Eye Plastic Surgery A Simplified Question And Answer Guide

Including My Ten Common Sense Rules For A Healthy Lifestyle

RONALD W. KRISTAN, MD FACS

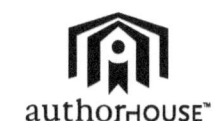

authorHOUSE™

1663 LIBERTY DRIVE, SUITE 200
BLOOMINGTON, INDIANA 47403
(800) 839-8640
WWW.AUTHORHOUSE.COM

AuthorHouse™
1663 Liberty Drive, Suite 200
Bloomington, IN 47403
www.authorhouse.com
Phone: 1-800-839-8640

AuthorHouse™ UK Ltd.
500 Avebury Boulevard
Central Milton Keynes, MK9 2BE
www.authorhouse.co.uk
Phone: 08001974150

©

First published by AuthorHouse 9/13/2006

ISBN: 1-4208-8031-4 (sc)
ISBN: 1-4208-8032-2 (dj)

Printed in the United States of America
Bloomington, Indiana

This book is printed on acid-free paper.

Dedicated to my family, Concetta, Jonathan, Stephen and Joseph for their love and support.

CONTENTS

PREFACE

I have written this book to educate the public about a specialty of medicine that is not well understood. After almost twenty years in the practice of ophthalmology with a subspecialty in eyelid plastic surgery, I became frustrated with continuing to have my patients ask, "where should I have my eyelid lift?". I have come to appreciate that most patients do not think of their "eye doctor" as someone who may be better trained to perform all aspects of eyelid surgery, including cosmetic eyelid "lifts". I am a plastic surgeon who has dedicated his entire career to only eyelid surgery. I have successfully performed thousands of eyelid operations.

The purpose of this book is not meant to establish a doctor-patient relationship or to constitute a second opinion. The content of this book is meant to be purely educational.

I hope that you find this book informative. I encourage any feedback you may have. Feel free to contact me at any of my offices or visit my website at DrKristan.com or eyeplastics.com

Ronald W. Kristan, MD FACS
180 White Road
Suite 202
Little Silver, NJ 07739
732-219-9220

279 Third Avenue
Suite 204
Long Branch, NJ 07740
732-222-7373

100 Commons Way
Suite 230
Holmdel, NJ 07733
732-796-7140

RONALD W. KRISTAN, MD FACS

BIOGRAPHY

Dr. Ronald W. Kristan is a Board Certified Physician and a Cosmetic Eyelid Rejuvenation Specialist. As a renowned eyelid plastic surgeon, Dr. Kristan is a leading specialist in this field with specific training, precision and experience to revitalize the highly delicate upper and lower eyelid areas. In fact, Dr. Kristan has successfully performed thousands of eyelid procedures. His innovative approach has resulted in the development of numerous new techniques that have been published. In fact, Dr. Kristan was instrumental in developing a laser procedure for tearing and was the first surgeon in the United States to perform the procedure. He has trained ophthalmologists from around the world in these techniques including Turkey, Italy and South America. He has published extensively and regularly presents papers at national and international meetings.

Additionally, Dr. Kristan employs laser facial rejuvenation to eliminate wrinkles and sun damaged skin. He also has extensive experience in the use of botulinum (botox) and utilizes this form of treatment for frown lines, forehead lines and crow's feet around the eyes.

Dr. Kristan graduated from New York University Medical School and completed his ophthalmology residency and subspecialty Fellowship in Ophthalmic Plastic and Reconstructive Surgery at Albany Medical Center. He is a Fellow of the prestigious American Society of Ophthalmic Plastic and Reconstructive Surgery as well as the American College of Surgeons. Dr. Kristan is one of five eye surgeons in New Jersey certified by the American Board of Eye Surgery in cataract and implant surgery. Dr. Kristan is listed in Who's Who in Medicine and Healthcare and has been voted one of the top eye plastic surgeons in New Jersey (New Jersey Life). Dr. Kristan is included in Castle Connolly's Listing of America's Cosmetic Doctors. Dr. Kristan is a Past President of the New Jersey Academy of Ophthalmology, where he is still an active member.

CHAPTER ONE

WHAT IS AN OCULOPLASTIC SURGEON AND WHAT DO THEY DO?

The specialty of Ophthalmic Plastic and Reconstructive Surgery actually had its origins in World War II. A group of physicians began to develop an interest in better understanding trauma to the eyelids and orbital (around the eye) area. These physicians were originally trained as eye surgeons. They felt whom better to treat and operate on the eyelids and periocular areas than those physicians most trained in eye surgery.

The culmination of their research and studies led to the formation of The American Society of Ophthalmic Plastic and Reconstructive Surgery (ASOPRS) in 1969. This organization embodies those of us that have advanced training and experience in this highly specialized field of eyelid and facial surgery. The eyelid tissue requires a through understanding of the unique anatomy. My eye surgery background is invaluable in this understanding.

To become a member of ASOPRS, I had to (1) study at an approved fellowship for one year (training beyond the required eye training); (2) sit for both written and oral board exams, and; (3) do original research and have it published. My original research was "The Use of the CO_2 Laser in Oculoplastic Surgery". I am very proud of this work which has been presented at national meetings.

Being an Oculoplastic surgeon allows me to specialize in all fields of eyelid and periocular surgery. I perform surgery for (1) aesthetic, cosmetic eyelid rejuvenation (eyelid lifts, botox and fillers/ restylane/collagen for wrinkles); (2) functional or malpositioned eyelids; (3) tumors of the eyelid, both benign and malignant, and; (4) tearing. Some tearing problems can be corrected without surgery, as can many eyelid conditions. Eyelid structures can be affected by normal aging changes, birth defects, injuries and inflammation. I have a special interest in dry eye, especially as it relates to the eyelids.

So as you can see, I belong to a very specialized group of physicians. In fact, there are only about 450 ASOPRS approved physicians nationally and internationally. This put me in a very elite group. I bring to my patients almost twenty years of experience in this field and feel uniquely qualified to handle all aspects of eyelid disorders and cosmetic eyelid surgery.

In general, I feel that more training and experience in an area does provide greater expertise. After graduating from medical school, I completed an internship, then three years of eye and eyelid surgery training, and one year specializing only in eyelid surgery. There is no other medical specialty that spends this much time training in eyelid surgery. Since many of the complications seen in eyelid surgery do affect the eyes, I feel that an oculoplastic surgeon is best trained to handle these problems. I have no desire to do cosmetic plastic surgery anywhere else in the body except the eyelids. I do not want to be an expert in everything. I have dedicated my entire career to this specialized area of functional and aesthetic eyelid surgery.

CHAPTER TWO

COSMETIC EYELID SURGERY

(BLEPHAROPLASTY)

What exactly is a blepharoplasty?
In simple terms, a blepharoplasty is an operation that removes excess tissue from the eyelids. Usually with the upper eyelids, surgery involves removal of excess skin with contouring of the eyelid crease. The lower eyelids often require the removal of puffy bags or redirecting the bags.

Sometimes filling in the depressions of the lower lid makes more sense. More on this in the chapter on fillers. It can be done for **functional** or **cosmetic** reasons. A functional baggy

Fig 1 This patient has overhanging eyelid tissue interfering with vision, a functional problem

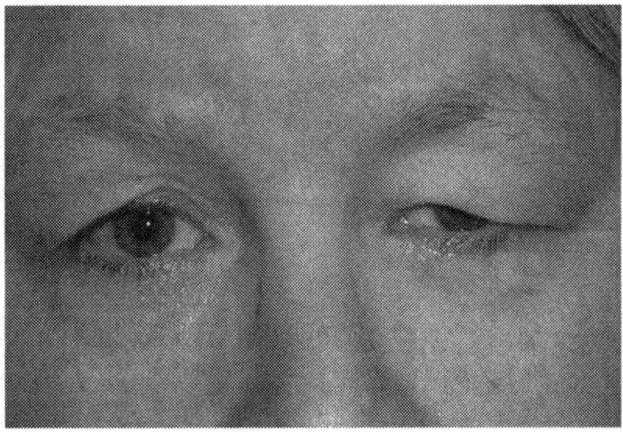

eyelid is called **dermatochalasis.** A **functional** blepharoplasty corrects overhanging eyelid tissue that is interfering with vision (Figure 1). Usually the peripheral vision is most affected. Patients with **functional** difficulties will often state that holding their eyelids up greatly improves vision. Lower eyelid surgery for removal of "bags" is always considered cosmetic (Figure 2). With lower eyelid cosmetic surgery the emphasis is on the "fat"- either to remove it or reposition it. Minimal removal of skin is usually indicated. This reduces the risk of the lower eyelid drooping after surgery (lid retraction-see below).

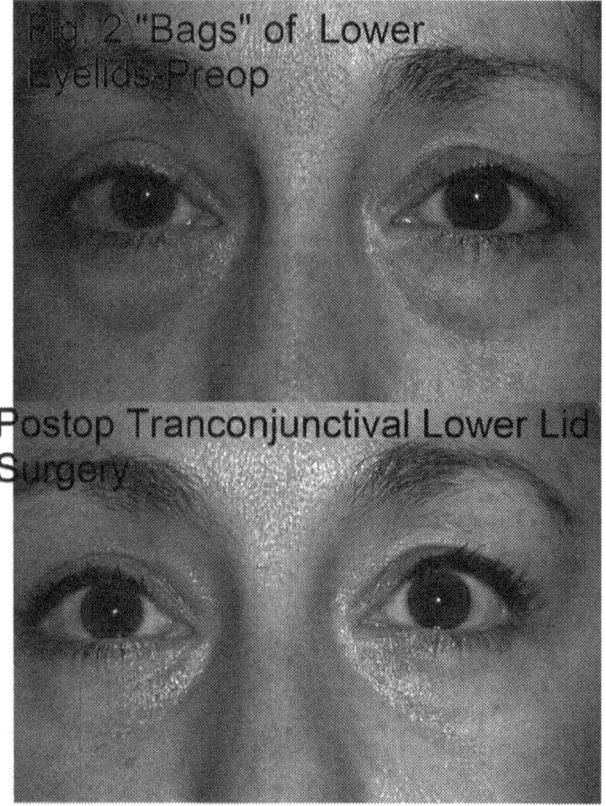

Fig. 2 "Bags" of Lower Eyelids-Preop

Postop Tranconjunctival Lower Lid Surgery

Cosmetic blepharoplasty is performed for an improved appearance. These patients are not having any difficulty with their vision. Aging and maturation of the face results in gravitational descent.

This causes the eyelids to sag and droop. I believe that heredity affects this process. I have had the opportunity to operate on three generations of the same family. Patients who elect to undergo cosmetic eyelid surgery want a refreshed and more youthful look. They want to reverse the aging process. This chapter will mostly be dedicated to a discussion of cosmetic eyelid surgery (Figure 3). I have found that most people having a blepharoplasty for functional reasons always seem to anticipate a certain cosmetic outcome. Remember that with a functional blepharoplasty the main complaint is related to loss of vision.

Why consider cosmetic eyelid surgery?
I believe that "your eyes" are the first thing people notice when they look at you. Your eyes reveal a lot about the way you feel. Sagging eyelids and puffy bags can make you look tired and older than you really are. Most patients feel their youthful and vibrant looking eyes have faded. They have tried many eye creams and cosmetics without results. Job situations may also prompt one to consider cosmetic eyelid surgery.

Remember that cosmetic eyelid surgery is a very personal decision.

What needs to be discussed before cosmetic eyelid surgery?
The best candidates for cosmetic eyelid surgery are men and women who are relatively healthy. There really is no age limit for these procedures. I feel that the preoperative consultation is most important. This is where I spend as much time as necessary to fully understand each patient's complaints and desires. **The most important thing that I emphasize during this visit is that patients have realistic goals and expectations. This will eliminate disappointment. Unhappy patients usually have unrealistic goals that were not understood preoperatively.** I have decided against operating on many patients because I felt that their goals were not realistic. I could not achieve these goals with surgery.

The decision to operate on both upper and lower eyelids is reviewed during this consultation.

Figure 3

BLEPHAROPLASTY

BEFORE   AFTER

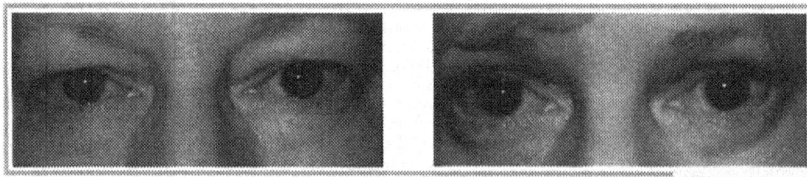

PATIENT A

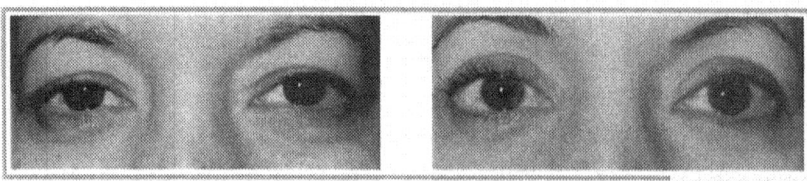

PATIENT B

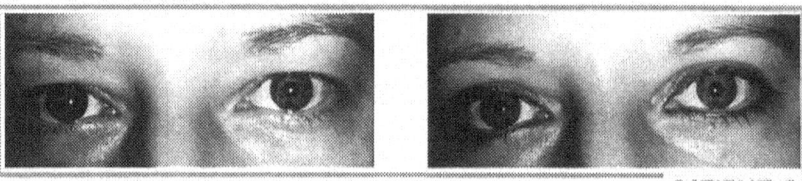

PATIENT C

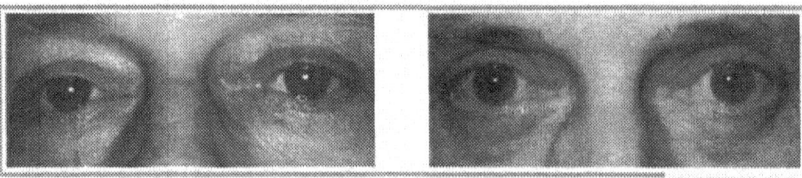

PATIENT D

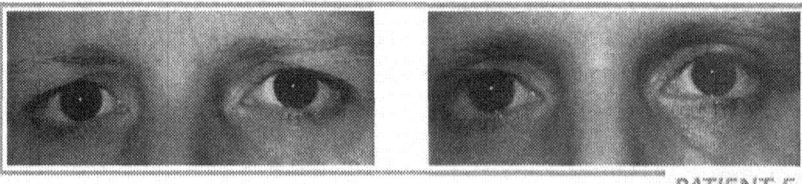

PATIENT E

BLEPHAROPLASTY

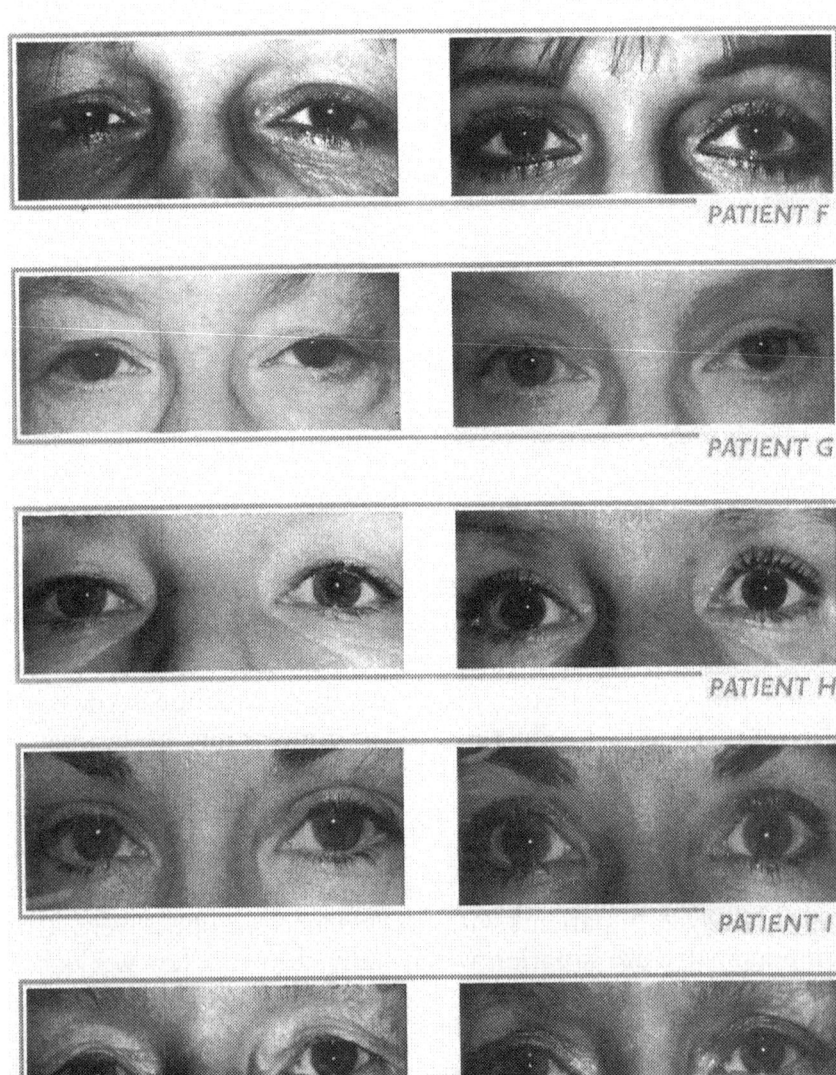

PATIENT F

PATIENT G

PATIENT H

PATIENT I

PATIENT J

BEFORE   AFTER

I can show you many pre and post-operative photos of patients that I have operated on. These are used only for illustration purposes and do not imply any guarantee. I also have many patients who would be happy to speak to you about their experience regarding the surgery and recovery process. Preoperative photographs are available for planning and discussion with the patient, intraoperative guidance, and postoperative comparison.

A complete history is imperative prior to any surgery. This includes:

1. Age
2. Medical history
3. Past surgeries
4. Ocular history
5. Family history
6. Social history
7. Medications
8. Allergies
9. Any bleeding tendencies

In addition, comprehensive eye and eyelid exams are performed. Since transient incomplete eyelid closure (lagophthalmos) is possible after surgery, tear production and stability must be evaluated preoperatively. With dry eye patients, I advise a more conservative approach to surgery. Lubricating drops and ointments may be needed in patients with dry eyes. Because eyelid surgery alters the blinking mechanism temporarily, a transient dry eye condition can result even in patients with no evidence pre-operatively. This temporary dry eye situation will usually clear in a few weeks but sometimes can take longer. Smoking is a major problem in anyone contemplating eyelid surgery. I believe it contributes to lax skin and definitely can affect the post-operative healing. I insist patients try and stop smoking prior to eyelid-especially cosmetic- surgery. Patients who continue to smoke after cosmetic eyelid surgery seem to regress faster than those that do not smoke.

Remember that blepharoplasty cannot get rid of wrinkles or crow's feet. Laser resurfacing, botox and fillers are used to address these problems. These procedures can, however, be performed at the same time as blepharoplasty. They will be discussed in more detail in Chapter 9.

What can I expect during and after surgery?

The surgery is performed in my state of the art ambulatory surgical center (ASC). This facility allows your surgery to be performed in the safest outpatient setting possible. Safety is always our utmost concern.

The actual surgical procedure can take anywhere from one to two hours depending on the number of eyelids being operated on. When you arrive at our ASC, my surgical team will begin to prepare you for surgery. They will ask you a number of questions and will start an intravenous (IV). This will allow us to administer medication to relax you. I will often take more photographs and we will discuss any last minute concerns that you might have. During the procedure, sedation is administered by my full time board certified anesthesiologist. This puts you in a comfortable, almost twilight state. I will make surgical marks on your eyelids with a special marking pen that guides me during the operation. Eye shields are placed into your eyes for protection. A surgical drape is used to keep the operative field sterile after your face is scrubbed with special soap. You feel no pain during the surgery. After surgery, you are usually in the recovery area for approximately 30 minutes.

Postoperative pain is usually minimal in my experience. Ice packs are immediately started for pain and swelling control. Swelling and black and blue (eccymosis) are maximum at about 48 hours and begin to diminish after this. Swelling and eccymosis usually fades during the first 1-2 weeks. I always tell patients that a certain amount of swelling can last 6 weeks to 6 months. The majority of patients, however, swelling is gone in the first few weeks. Most people return to their normal routine after the first week. The stitches are removed in 7-10 days. I have seen persistent swelling in patients with thyroid disease. This is carefully reviewed preoperatively in all patients with known thyroid disease contemplating cosmetic eyelid surgery.

Table 1 reviews my postoperative instructions.

TABLE 1

INSTRUCTIONS FOR CARE AFTER EYELID SURGERY

1. **Expect some swelling and bruising of the eyelids. Everyone reacts differently but most swelling/bruising will likely be gone in 1 to 2 weeks. Swelling and bruising are very unpredictable with some patients barely swelling while others bruise significantly. As mentioned about the final outcome may not become apparent for 6 weeks to 6 months. There is no way to know this before surgery assuming all blood thinning medications have been appropriately stopped. For the first week avoid dusty situations. Use common sense regarding strenuous activities, especially outside. You may want to wear sunglasses.**

2. **You may wash your hair and bathe but do not scrub over the operated area or get soap in your eyes. If the operated area gets wet, gently pat dry with a clean towel. Do not use any ointment, drops or medication other than those directed by the doctor. All glaucoma medications should be continued. All other medications for blood pressure, diabetes and any heart condition should be used based on instructions from your medical doctor. If you have stopped blood thinners, like coumadin, this will most likely be started right after surgery. This will be discussed with you post-operatively.**

3. **Do not use eyelid makeup or swim for at least 3 weeks after surgery or as directed by Dr. Kristan**

4. DO NOT RUB THE OPERATED EYE. Mucus and tears can be gently cleaned from the lids with warm water and clean tissues. Do this also if the lids are stuck together. Always wash your hands before administering medications or touching the operative area.

5. Ice packs should be used for the first 24 hours. I recommend using frozen peas in freezer bags applied for 10-15 minutes on and 10-15 minutes off. Do not sleep with the ice packs (there is a remote risk of frost bite with ice on the lids for all that time). Avoid strenuous activity of all kinds including bending at the waist during the first 24 hours. It would also be helpful if you can sleep with your head slightly elevated for the first 24 hours. This helps with the swelling. If you do not have a patch, check vision by covering each eye and read the newspaper. You may have to blink to clear the vision as the ointment can interfere with seeing.

6. Most pain can be controlled with regular or extra strength Tylenol (acetaminophen). AVOID ASPIRIN. If you are having severe pain that is not controlled call the office immediately.

7. If an eye patch was applied, you will be instructed on when to remove it. There may be some oozing of blood and mucus from the wounds or through the patch. This is normal. IF BLEEDING IS CONTINUOUS APPLY MILD PRESSURE TO THE EYE. IF THE BLEEDING DOES NOT STOP, CALL THE OFFICE IMMEDIATELY.

8. Medications can include ointment and/or drops for the affected eye(s) and oral medication. Dr. Kristan or one of my nurses will instruct you in their use.

9. Warm compresses can be applied to the area on the third day after surgery using a washcloth. Water can be heated up in the microwave or boiled. REMEMBER TO TEST THE WATER FIRST SO THAT IT IS NOT TOO HOT!

10. Lubricating drops/ointments may be necessary in the post-operative period to help with mucus discharge, sticky eyelids, and transient dry eyes. Topical tear drops come in both a preservative and non-preservative formula. The preservative formula usually comes in a larger bottle. Because the preservatives can be irritating, I usually recommend the non-preservative drops. These come in a single dose, disposable vials. Almost all of the common brands (refresh, cellufresh, theratears, and gen teal) come in preservative free dosing. In addition, sometimes a more viscous tear drop supplement is necessary, like celluvisc. For morning problems related to dry eyes, I will frequently recommend a lubricating ointment at bedtime. Common brands include refresh PM and lacrilube.

11. Dr. Kristan will discuss returning to work with you, if applicable. If you are unsure about your instructions or have any questions as to your surgery or aftercare, do not hesitate to call.

What are risks and complications associated with cosmetic eyelid surgery?
Like any surgical procedure, risks and complications are possible. **Table 2** illustrates the form I review with every patient as part of my informed consent. In summary, some of the potential complications of blepharoplasty include: eyelid crease scar, cysts, under correction, inability to close the eye, asymmetry, high eyelid crease, sunken eye, droopy eyelid, infection, decrease or loss of vision, hemorrhage (bleeding), numbness of eyelids, retraction or frank ectropion (pulling down of the lower eyelid), and double vision (diplopia).

Who should perform your surgery?
There are many physicians trained in cosmetic surgery. As I've stated elsewhere in this book, I am specifically trained as an eyelid cosmetic surgeon. Experience is very important. I have been doing

cosmetic eyelid surgery since 1984. I have performed over 5,000 eyelid surgeries in my career. I have developed my own personal philosophy regarding cosmetic eyelid surgery and the "youthful eyelid" that I would be happy to share with you. This comes from performing and studying thousands of my results and the results of others. Most importantly, you need to develop a trusting relationship with your surgeon who listens to your concerns and is easy to talk to.

TABLE 2

DISCUSSION I HAVE WITH EVERY PATIENT PRIOR TO SURGERY

As per the patients' request, a blepharoplasty operation has been discussed in detail. The patient clearly understands and accepts the following:

- As in any cosmetic/functional procedure, the goal of surgery is improvement not perfection

- The final result may not be apparent for months post-op. Cosmetic surgery is an on going process of treatment, enhancement, stabilization and healing

- In order to achieve the best possible result, more than one procedure may be required

- Strict adherence to the post-op regimen is necessary in order to achieve the best result

I have discussed with the patient multiple techniques for performing upper and/or lower eyelid blepharoplasty. I will always individualize which approach to use to assure the best possible outcome. These include but are not limited to:

- Incisions with standard surgical blades

- Incisions using lasers

- Incisions using radiofrequency

- Transconjunctival incision for the lower eyelid. This incision involves going behind the eyelid thus avoiding an external incision and potential scar. My training as an eye surgeon makes me very comfortable with this approach since one is operating very close to the eyeball with this technique

The patient understands that the following complications are possible from blepharoplasty surgery by any technique. These include but are not limited to:

- Bleeding: in order to avoid potentially serious bleeding all medications that can "thin the blood" are stopped well in advance of surgery. These include vitamin E, any medication with aspirin, and Advil or Motrin. Also many herbal supplements such a ginkgo biloba used for improved memory and cardiovascular status, can result in an increased bleeding tendency. My surgical counselor will review this carefully with you before surgery.

- Infection

- Under correction or over correction

- Objectionable scarring is rare but can occur: patients will often feel tightness after surgery. This almost always resolves over time and may take up to 6 months

- Alteration of skin pigmentation. This is usually temporary, but rarely can be permanent

- Lower eyelid retraction: this happens if surgery is too aggressive on the lower eyelids and scar tissue develops-usually resolves with time but sometimes needs surgical repair. I have fortunately never had this complication happen to me

- Double vision: this is rare and usually transient. Double vision occurs because of scarring of the extraocular muscles (the muscles that surround the eye). I have only seen this happen once in 20 years and it was not on a patient that I operated on.

- Dry eye: this was discussed above

- Change in the shape of the eye: usually this happens if too much tissue is removed, that is, a more aggressive blepharoplasty

- Inability to completely close the eye

- Persistent swelling: I see this more frequently in patients with thyroid disease

- Transient numbness in the upper lid: I see this very frequently and have never seen it persist more than a few months

Each of these potential problems is reviewed as to why they may occur and how often.

I usually close the discussion with the following comments:

- The patient's questions were answered and the patient seemed to have a clear understanding of what was discussed. Patient has had the opportunity to ask any questions. Alternatives to blepharoplasty such as accepting present condition have been discussed. No guarantee as to outcome was suggested to the patient.

Although this is a more specific format for a blepharoplasty operation, I use a similar approach for giving informed consent for all surgeries that I perform. I believe that it is important for patients to fully understand all of the risks involved with any operation, the usual surgical experience and the post operative course. Most patients are naturally apprehensive about surgery. This pre-operative counseling makes for a more educated patient, allaying many of their tensions. Avoiding complications and carefully dealing with complications is paramount in any surgical experience. If problems do occur after surgery, they can usually be overcome with surgeon and patient working closely together in a caring and reassuring way.

CHAPTER THREE

UPPER EYELID DROOPING (PTOSIS)

What is ptosis?
Ptosis is a condition of the upper eyelid that causes it to droop (Figure 4). The eyelid margin (the area of the eyelid where the eyelashes come out of) hangs down in front of the pupil (black opening) of the eye. The pupil is the window into the eye—like a window in your house. The pupil allows the images from the outside world to enter your eye. If the upper eyelid margin is lower than it should be and blocks the pupil, ptosis results. As a result, ptosis can interfere with your vision. Ptosis is one of the most common lid problems that I see.

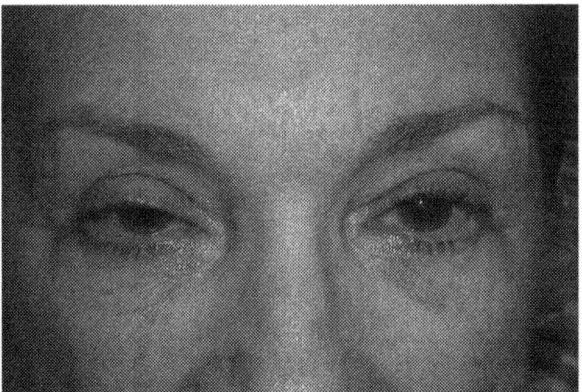

Fig 4. Notice than in this patient the upper eyelid margin covers the eye, moreso on the right. The upper lid is blocking this person's vision

What are the symptoms and signs of ptosis?

As can be inferred from above, visual complaints are the most common symptoms of ptosis. These can range from loss of peripheral vision to difficulty reading. Many patients with ptosis complain of "tired eyes". Patients will often complain that they have to "hold their eyelids up in order to see". Sustained reading also becomes very difficult with ptosis of the upper eyelid. A number of measurements are made in diagnosing ptosis of the upper eyelid. These include the eyelid crease height, the levator function and the margin reflex distance or MRD. The eyelid crease is measured from the lid margin to the eyelid skin crease. The levator function is measured by having the patient look from a down position to an up gaze position while immobilizing the brow. The MRD measures the distance from the middle of the pupil to the upper eyelid margin.

Is ptosis different from baggy eyelids (dermatochalasis)?

Baggy upper eyelids (dermatochalasis) are different from ptosis. With baggy upper eyelids the lid margin is in a normal position-unlike ptosis. Baggy eyelids describe a condition of the upper lids caused by excess skin that hangs over the lid. The symptoms of baggy eyelids and ptosis, however, can be very similar. Both interfere with vision as described above. Treatment involves a different type of operation. **Dermatochalasis** is what most people refer to as aging of the upper eyelid (see figure 1, chapter two). Dermatochalasis can also occur as the brow begins to descend worsening the redundant skin and muscle of the upper lid skin fold. An oculoplastic surgeon can easily make this distinction.

What are the causes of ptosis?

Ptosis is broken down into a congenital form (present from birth) and an acquired form. A third form called myogenic ptosis is usually inherited, caused by a primary muscle abnormality. Myogenic ptosis makes up a very small part of the ptosis cases I see. Usually in myogenic ptosis there is a progressive wasting of the muscle. The acquired form can occur at any age, but typically occurs after the age of 60. Most cases of ptosis are caused by a defect in the muscle that raises and lowers the upper eyelid called the **levator muscle**. Let's talk briefly about the muscles involved with opening and closing the eyes.

As mentioned above, the muscle in the upper eyelid that raises the lid is called the **levator muscle.** There is a separate muscle that surrounds the eye in both the upper and lower eyelid called the **orbicularis muscle** that closes the eye. Thus the levator muscle allows the eye to open and the orbicularis muscle causes the eye to close. There is fat between the orbicularis muscle and the levator muscle that acts as a shock absorber and allows for smooth movement of the eyelid. So if you really think about it, the blink reflex is a very complicated interplay between these two muscles. An additional muscle called **Muller's muscle** is responsible for an involuntary elevation in the upper eyelid and is affected by different hormonal levels in the body.

In congenital cases, the levator muscle does not form properly. The levator function will always be reduced. In the acquired cases, the muscle functioned normally prior to the onset of the ptosis. For some unknown reason, the levator muscle stretches and weakens over time causing the eyelid to drop. The levator muscle, however, in acquired ptosis still has good to excellent function. Possible causes of levator weakening includes (1) previous surgery, (2) eyelid swelling secondary to infection or allergies, (3) manipulation and stretching of the eyelid from contact lens use, and (4) trauma to the eye area.

There are some neurological conditions that can cause ptosis, such as myasthenia gravis. Other neurologic disorders include third cranial nerve palsies, Horner syndrome, multiple sclerosis and ophthalmoplegic migraine. Your history and physical exam can provide clues to a possible neurological etiology, such as unequal pupils, orbital inflammation, double vision and abnormal facial spasms. A neurology consultation and brain scan may be necessary.

What are the treatments for ptosis of the upper eyelid?
If the ptosis is caused by certain neurological conditions, medicine may elevate the eyelid. If the ptosis is mild enough and there are

no real symptoms, the condition can be followed conservatively with no treatment. If symptomatic with visual difficulties, ptosis is corrected by surgery. Surgery may be modified if factors such as dry eye, Bell's palsy, scarring of the eyelid, or an inability to close the lid are present.

What type of surgery is done for ptosis?

Congenital Ptosis: Surgery is usually postponed until age 3-4 unless the ptosis is severe enough to be causing a lazy eye and permanent visual loss. Surgery is aimed at strengthening the weak and malformed levator muscle. Sometimes the levator is so weak that the brow muscles must be used in the surgical correction. Out of all the ptosis surgery I do, I find congenital ptosis to be the most challenging and difficult to achieve consistently excellent results.

Acquired ptosis: Surgery to strengthen the levator muscle is my preferred choice to correct ptosis. Some surgeons will elevate the eyelid by tightening the posterior (back) tissues of the eyelid. This technique is equally as effective. The majority of ptosis repair that I perform is for the acquired type.

What can I expect after the surgery?

Usually the eyelid will remain swollen for one to two weeks. In addition, varying amounts of "black and blue" will be present. Pain is minimal for the first 24 hours. I have my patient return to their full activity level as soon as they feel up to it. This is usually after 48 hours. The incision sites are treated with ointments. The stitches come out in one week. Most people complain that the eyelids feel a little tight and numb for a few days. These feelings almost always disappear. It is typical for the eyelid height to fluctuate during the first few weeks.

What are the complications of ptosis surgery?

As with other eyelid surgery, bleeding and infection are risks. In addition, ptosis surgery can result in an under correction about 5-10% of the time. This means that the procedure may need to be repeated either with the same or a different technique. Over corrections can occur as well. Fortunately over corrections are much less common. They are also more difficult to fix. If only one eyelid is operated on an interesting phenomenon called Herrings' Law may make the unoperated upper eye drop after surgery even though nothing was done to that lid. This is discussed in detail pre-operatively and testing can be performed to see if this will happen. It is often unpredictable, however, and we need to always be prepared that the unoperated eye may drop. Fortunately, this can be fixed with another ptosis operation on the other upper eyelid.

Does my insurance cover ptosis surgery?

Most insurance companies have criterion that determines whether ptosis surgery will be covered. Usually your insurance company will require precertification. My staff will take care of this. Medicare is the exception. They do not do precertifications.

If dermatochalasis is also present, can it be corrected at the same time as a ptosis repair?

Dermatochalasis (baggy eyelids) can be corrected at the same time as a ptosis repair. Your insurance company may consider it to be cosmetic, however, and not covered for payment. Dermatochalasis surgery would then be treated as a cosmetic procedure.

CHAPTER FOUR

ENTROPION (EYELID TURNING IN)

What is an Entropion?

An entropion is a degenerative condition that causes the eyelid to rotate inward (Figure 5). This can be congenital in nature, which means you are born with it. Congenital entropion is rare. More commonly, entropion occurs in the aging eyelid. I like to call this involutional entropion. Most people with involutional entropion are over the age of 65. Entropion can occur in the upper eyelid but most of the time involves the lower eyelid. Entropion can involve one eyelid or two (Figure 6).

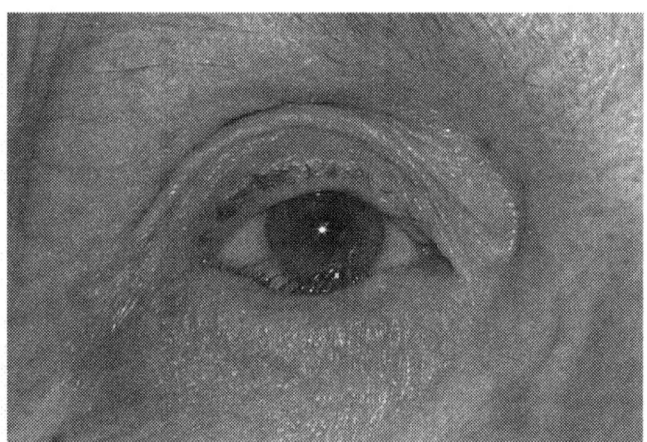

Fig. 5 Notice the lower eyelid is rotated inward with the eyelashes scratching the eyeball

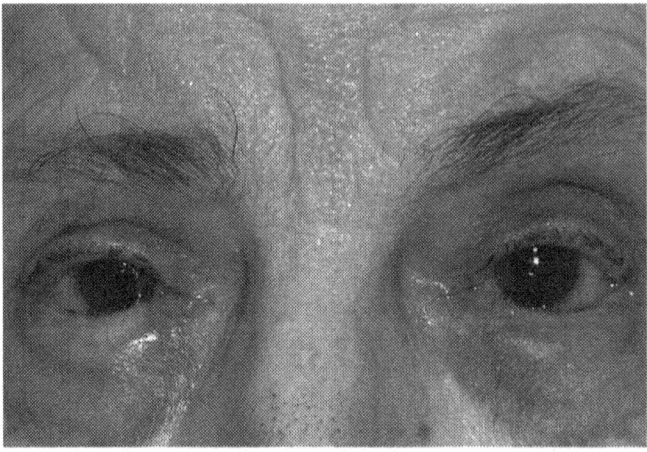

Fig. 6 Entropion involving both lower eyelids

What causes an entropion?
Since most cases of entropion involve the lower eyelid in our older population, my discussion will be restricted to this category. This type is called **involutional entropion.**

If you think about a hammock that is suspended at its' two ends, the lower eyelid is very similar. The inner end and outer end of the lower eyelid are attached to the nasal bone (inner) and orbital bone (outer), just like a hammock. This allows the eyelid to rotate, just like a hammock. If you have ever tried getting into a hammock, you know how easy it rotates. During youth, the eyelid is firm enough to resist this rotation and stays in place. As we age, however, the lower eyelid tissues become more lax and stretch. This allows the eyelid to easily rotate. An entropion results when the particular stabilizing structures of the eyelid undergo this aging/degenerative process. Another less common type of entropion is called **cicatricial entropion.** This is caused by scarring of the inner part of the eyelid causing the entire eyelid to turn in.

Why doesn't everyone over the age of 65 develop an entropion?
As long as the structures required for stabilization remain intact, an entropion will not develop. There is no way to predict who will develop an entropion.

Are there any other medical conditions that predispose one to the development of an entropion, like diabetes or hypertension?
Not to my knowledge

What are the symptoms of a lower eyelid entropion?
The most common symptoms of a lower eyelid entropion are redness and a scratchy eye. This is a very uncomfortable condition. Just think about how painful it can be having one eyelash stuck in the eye. With an entropion, the whole row of lower lashes is hitting the eye.

Most patients with entropion are not aware the eyelid is turning in. They just know their eye is irritated and always feels like "something is in it". If the eye gets scratched, an infection can ensue.

Most of the patients I see for this condition are referred in by other physicians because of my expertise in this field.

What can be done to correct an entropion?
Entropion correction requires surgery. Rarely have I used BOTOX as a treatment for entropion. This is, however, only a temporary measure. There is no medicine that fixes this problem. (Figure 6a)

Pre op entropion lower lid   Lower eyelid in normal position after surgery

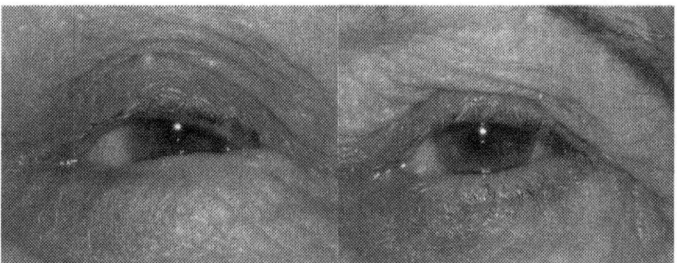

Can you tell me about the surgery?

Surgery is done in an outpatient setting under local anesthesia. It usually takes about 30 minutes for the entire procedure. Sedation is administered so you are very comfortable and don't feel anything. The eyelid weakness is repaired and stabilized. Frequently the eye is patched overnight. The patch is removed the following day and ointment is used. Most patients return to their normal activity the next day.

For cicatricial entropion, surgery is a little more complicated and frequently will require a skin graft and patching for a few days.

Are there any complications from the surgery?

Like any surgery, there can be complications. The two most common complications are bleeding and infection. Fortunately, infection is uncommon. Bleeding causes "black and blue" resulting in a "black eye". This "shiner" disappears in one to two weeks and has no adverse effect on the outcome of the surgery.

Can an entropion come back after surgery is done?

I have a 95% success rate correcting involutional entropion. One can not predict who will recur or who will need more than one procedure. Fortunately, in my hands, this doesn't happen too often. Cicatricial entropion has a higher rate of recurrence and may require more than one operation.

Are there any other eyelid conditions that cause the eyelashes to rub against the eye?

The three most common lash problems include **cicatricial entropion (discussed above), trichiasis, and acquired distichiasis.** With trichiasis and distichiasis, the eyelid margin is not turned in. The eyelid is in a normal position but the eyelashes are misdirected, hitting the eye. These conditions usually result from eyelid inflammation that causes scarring within the eyelid. These eyelash disorders can be managed either by (1) repeated epilation (pulling the eyelashes out in the office), (2) destruction or removal of offending lashes and their follicles (electrolysis or cryo/freezing), or (3) surgical alteration of the eyelid.

CHAPTER FIVE

ECTROPION (EYELID TURNING OUT)

What is an ectropion?
An ectropion is a degenerative condition that causes the eyelid to rotate out and away from the eyeball (Figure 7). It usually occurs over the age of 65. Think of an ectropion as the opposite of an entropion we discussed in chapter four.

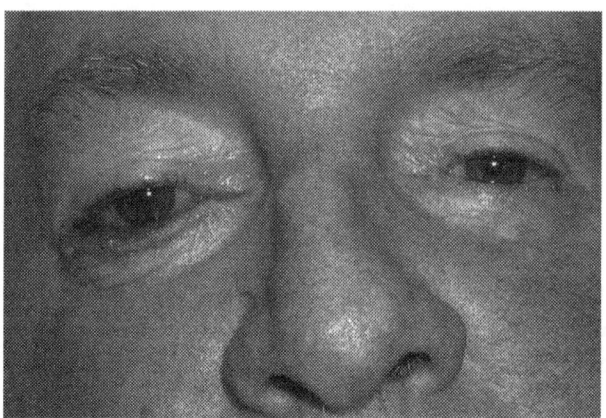

Fig 7. Notice the severe irritation caused by an ectropion of the lower eyelid

What causes an ectropion?
Just like in an entropion, laxity and weakness in the lower eyelid predispose to the development of an ectropion. As gravity causes the midface to descend over time, eyelid weakness and

poor support can result in the lower eyelid turning out. Again, there is no way to predict who will develop an ectropion (Figure 8). The most common form of ectropion is called **involutional ectropion** caused by this eyelid laxity. **Cicatricial ectropion** occurs when there is scarring in the eyelid skin shortening the eyelid and turning it out. **Paralytic ectropion** usually is caused by an orbicularis muscle weakness of the lower lid commonly seen after a Bell's palsy.

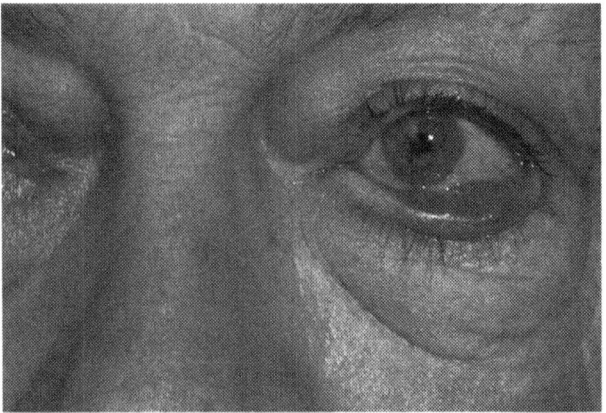

Fig 8. Severe ectropion of the lower eyelid

Are there any other medical conditions that predispose one to the development of an ectropion?

Some skin conditions, such as rosacea, can cause certain types of ectropion. Also, inflammatory eyelid conditions, such as blepharitis, have been implicated. An **interesting** condition that I consider to be a subset of ectropion is **floppy eyelid syndrome.** Floppy eyelid syndrome occurs because of a degenerative disorder of the tarsus or eyelid support system. This results in the upper eyelid everting usually at night during sleep. Symptoms include chronic discharge-especially in the morning- irritation and tearing. These patients are usually overweight and have sleep apnea (difficulty falling asleep or waking up frequently). In addition to the eyelid management, their other medical problems need to be carefully addressed by their medical specialists.

What are the symptoms of a lower eyelid ectropion?
The most common symptoms of a lower eyelid ectropion are redness, tearing and irritation. The eye usually has a mucous discharge. The exposed part of the eyelid gets very red and dry. Crusting on this exposed part of the eyelid can develop and dry up. The biggest risk with an ectropion of the lower eyelid is drying of the eye and infection (Figure 9).

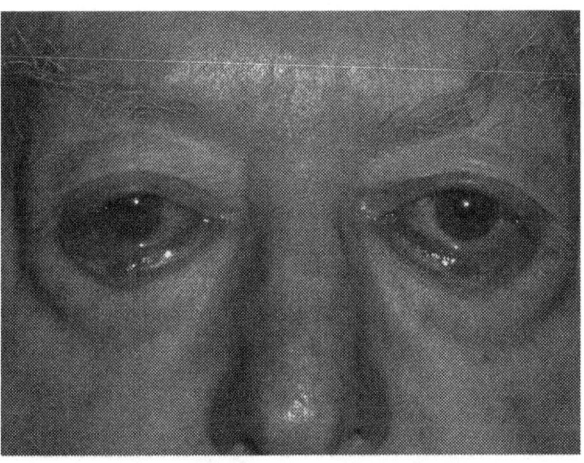

Fig 9. Ectropion of both lower eyelids causing dryness, crusting and infection

What is done to correct an ectropion?
Initially, one might try eye ointments to quiet down the inflammation and redness. A small number of ectropions may respond to this therapy only. However the majority of lower eyelid ectropions need to be repaired surgically.

Can you describe the surgical repair of an ectropion?
Surgery is performed in our outpatient surgical suite under local anesthesia with sedation. The procedure can take from

30 minutes to one hour, depending on the complexity of the correction. Most of the time the eyelid is corrected by a tightening procedure. This applies to all forms of ectropion. Sometimes a skin graft is necessary, especially with cicatricial ectropion. This is usually taken from the upper eyelid or from behind the ear. Patching is almost always required. Sometimes the eyelid is stitched closed for a few days. Fortunately there is minimal pain, even with the more involved cases. The surgical complications are the usual ones for eyelid surgery, including bleeding and infection. If a skin graft is placed, there is a small chance that it may not take. This does not happen too often. Because the eyelids are very vascularized (have a lot of blood vessels), skin grafts have an excellent chance for survival.

Recovery can take one to six weeks depending on whether a skin graft was placed or not. None of these procedures usually interfere with getting back to your normal routine as soon as possible.

Treatment of floppy eyelid syndrome is both with lubricating ointments and shielding/patching the eye at night. A surgical procedure is frequently needed in addition to shortening the length of the eyelid.

Do ectropions recur?
Unfortunately ectropions can recur. If due to chronic inflammatory skin conditions, the process will continue despite an excellent and successful surgical repair. All attempts are made to aggressively treat all chronic skin ailments. Sometimes this is done in conjunction with a dermatologist.

Eyelid malpositions can also occur in children. Ptosis, entropion, ectropion can be seen on a congenital (from birth) basis. Management needs to be individualized because of some special situations unique to children. For instance, ptosis in a child could result in a lazy eye (amblyopia) if the eyelid covers the visual axis during the first decade of life. Surgery for ptosis may need to be performed to prevent this. Other eyelid conditions in children are managed based on symptoms and with the goal of excellent visual development. Surgical repair will usually require general anesthesia.

CHAPTER SIX

WHY DOES MY EYE WATER

OR TEAR ALL THE TIME?

Can anything be done for my tearing?
Tearing is a condition that can be very annoying and frustrating. Usually tearing does not represent a serious problem. Tearing can interfere with vision in many situations. Visual difficulties and embarrassment from constant wiping of tears are what prompt most people to consult with me for relief. Most of the time tearing can be improved, if not cured. I will usually ask how symptomatic patients are from the tearing. This will dictate what course of treatment is considered.

The tear film is a very complex surface consisting of a **mucin (mucus) layer, an oil layer and an aqueous (water) layer.** Mucin is produced by tiny cells in the conjunctiva called **goblet cells.** Oils are secreted by **meibomian glands** located in the eyelids. The water component of the tears comes from the **lacrimal** gland located under the upper eyelid in the outer corner (known as the temporal area).All three of these layers must be healthy for the eye to function properly. Evaluation of the tear film must always be considered in looking for a cause of tearing.

What are the causes of tearing?
I like to think of the causes of tearing as threefold. One is that too many tears are produced (hypersecretion). Second that the tears are distributed in an abnormal way and third, that the tears can't drain fast enough (excretory outflow obstruction). As mentioned above, the aqueous layer of tears is made in a gland located in the

upper outer area under the eyelid (Figure A). The blinking action of the eyelids then distributes the tears over the surface of the eye and pushes them to the inner corner where the tear duct drain is located. There are two openings in the eyelids that drain tears, one in the upper and one in the lower eyelid. The lower eyelid probably drains most of the tears. The tears eventually drain down into the nose. That's why you can sometimes taste your eye drops after instillation.

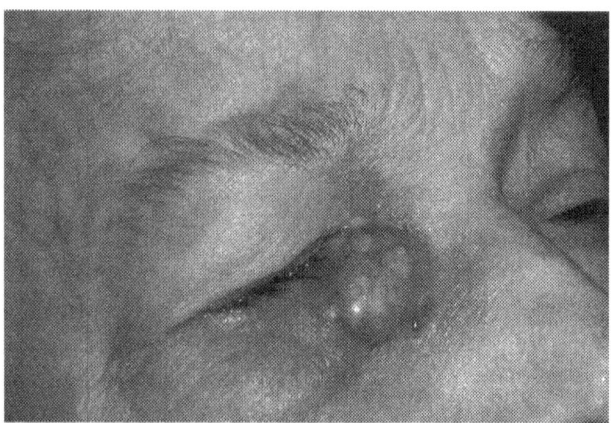

Fig 10. This patient has a blockage in her tear duct causing a severe infection.

What causes too many tears to be produced?
This is usually caused by external factors. Situations such as the cold or wind can cause more tears to be produced. Allergies are a very common cause of excessive tear production. Certain eyelid inflammation such as blepharitis results in tearing. Any acute eye infection or inflammation results in the eye trying to lubricate itself and tears are produced in excess.

Interestingly, dry eyes can result in excessive tear production. That's right! Dry eyes are actually a cause of tearing. How could this be, you ask? When your eyes are dry the brain senses this dryness through a reflex mechanism. As far as the brain is concerned, more tears need to be produced. Because the brain is the ultimate organ controlling tear production, a signal is sent to the tear glands to make more tears. If the tear duct drains can not handle the excess tearing will be the symptom. So believe it or not, sometimes the treatment for tearing is to use moisture drops or wetting drops.

What causes tears not to drain properly?

The most common cause of decreased drainage of tears through the tear duct drain is an obstruction (Figure 10). This can be the result of aging changes, trauma, scarring, inflammation, and the use of certain medication. Both topical and systemic medications can cause scarring of the tear duct.

Certain chemotherapeutic drugs for cancer treatment can cause structural changes to the tear duct resulting in narrowing and loss of outflow.

In addition, laxity of eyelid tissue seen with aging can result in decrease of the pumping action of the lower eyelid. Every time the eyelid blinks, the lower eyelid moves back and forth pushing the tears into the tear duct drain. If the lower eyelid does not properly perform this task, the tears will roll over the top of the lower eyelid. Correcting these structural problems will usually improve the tearing.

How is the cause of tearing determined?

Evaluation of tearing requires a comprehensive eye exam. Vision, external exam, tear film, eyelid exam, blink mechanism and the inside of the eye are all carefully checked. Mechanical irritation of the eye can be caused by an ectropion (turning out of the lid), entropion (turning in of the lid) or trichiasis (abnormal eyelashes). Next, I evaluate whether there is a structural defect in the drainage system. There may be a blockage in the tear duct system right at the opening-referred to as **punctal stenosis.** The tear duct drain is evaluated by probing and irrigating the drain. This is a simple office procedure, but tells me if an obstruction is present and where it is. And remember from a previous question that an exam for testing for dry eyes must be performed. After this evaluation, a treatment plan is formulated. Pertinent history should also include sinus disease, nasal surgery, trauma, allergies, and topical medications (eye drops). Also it is necessary to know if the patient has been on chemotherapy as mentioned above. In some patients, more advanced testing may be necessary. This usually includes some form of radiology such as an MRI scan or a CT scan. In specific instances, these tests may be combined with injection of a radio opaque dye in to the tear drain to rule out a suspected tumor.

What treatments are available for the correction of tearing?
In some situations, tearing can not be completely cured. Most patients who are significantly bothered by tearing will be happy with any improvement.

If the eyes are found to be dry or there is an alteration in the ocular surface, I will first begin dry eye/ocular surface disease therapy. This may involve modifying ones' environment, tear supplements, vitamins and the use of a new drop that actually helps make new tears called **restasis.** Most external inflammations such as allergies can be treated with combination drops and antihistamine medications, including nasal sprays. Sometimes a referral to an allergist may be necessary. Other eyelid inflammations-most commonly **blepharitis**- are usually treated with drops and ointments.

If eyelid malpositions are found, these are usually corrected with various surgical procedures. These procedures can range from simple lid tightened techniques with one stitch to more complex surgeries. Most of these can be done in our ambulatory surgical center right in our office.

If the tear duct drain is found to be obstructed, treatment usually involves a surgical repair. Again, depending on where the obstruction is, the surgery can be rather simple or more complex. The latter procedures often involve admission to the hospital for outpatient surgery. Some techniques involve inserting flexible tubes within the tear duct drain. Others involve creating a new drain into the nose. Still others involve bypassing the normal drain altogether and having the tears drain into the nose through a glass tube. This tube is completely concealed. It has been used for almost thirty years with excellent results and safety.

I have also cured many tearing patients by simply irrigating the tear duct. I believe that some patients may form a small stone in the duct that I am able to flush out. Periodic flushing helps prevent tearing from recurring.

Can tearing occur in children?
The simple answer is yes, but sometimes requires a different approach. Let me explain. It is not uncommon for many newborns to tear. This is because the tear duct drain (Figure A) fully opens up somewhere between 36-40 weeks of gestation (the development of the newborn). Since most infants are born during this time, it is not unusual to have tearing and/or frank infection at birth. My approach to these infants is to do a careful eye exam to make sure there is no other eye disease present. These children are watched carefully.

Fortunately, most of the tearing resolves in the first few months. If not resolved by about one year, I will usually recommend a surgical procedure to open up the tear duct drain. Sometimes repeated infections may necessitate operating sooner. Other than a congenital origin, tearing in children is usually caused by some external process-like allergy- similar to the discussion above.

So you see that tearing involves a very detailed and comprehensive evaluation. Most of the time tearing can be significantly improved, if not cured. Some of my happiest patients are those that I have helped with tearing.

CHAPTER SEVEN

WHAT IS A BELL'S PALSY (FACIAL DROOP)?

What Is a Bell's palsy?

A Bell's palsy is a weakness of one of the cranial (brain) nerves causing the face to droop. The nerve involved is the seventh cranial nerve. The seventh cranial nerve controls all of the facial muscles. Besides helping the eyes and mouth close, these muscles are important in maintaining facial expressions (Figure 11).

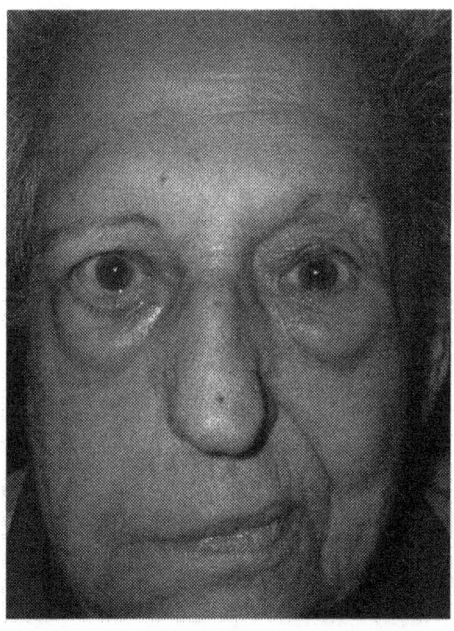

Fig 11. Patient with right facial droop

What are the causes of a Bell's palsy?

The most common cause of a facial droop is usually a viral infection. The actual virus is rarely isolated. Technically this is very difficult to do. Most facial palsies due to a viral infection usually resolve over a few months. Herpes simplex virus can produce a characteristic Bell's palsy and can be treated with oral medication (acyclovir, famvir or valtrex).

Some of the more serious causes include a stroke, brain tumor, and parotid gland tumor (a salivary gland just in front of the ear). In addition some patients with Lyme disease or facial trauma can present with a seventh nerve palsy.

Sometimes, a facial palsy can result from surgery to remove various tumors. Usually these involve a specific area of the brain or the parotid gland.

How can I recognize a Bell's palsy?

People with a Bell's palsy have a characteristic asymmetry in their face. They look like they have had a stroke. The lip droops, as do all the facial muscles on the involved side. The brow is lower and the eyelid has difficulty closing. Most people will notice difficulty in speaking. This is what usually first alerts most patients that something is wrong. Onset is usually acute; that is happens rather quickly.

What should I do if I recognize these symptoms?

I consider a facial palsy to be a medical emergency. Depending on your age, your doctor needs to make sure that you are not having a stroke. Some strokes can be reversed if caught early enough. Your regular doctor first assesses and treats all Bell's palsies, not an oculoplastic specialist. A neurologist is frequently involved through consultation.

A work-up usually consists of an extensive history, brain and parotid gland scans, extensive blood work, and complete neurological physical exam.

Is there treatment for a Bell's palsy?
Depending on the cause treatment may be available. Clearly if a treatable infection is found like lyme disease, antibiotics can be used.

If a stroke is found, then careful assessment for clot dissolving medications needs to be made. This is usually done in the emergency room by the stroke team. For unknown viral infections, corticosteroids are sometimes used.

**What is the role of an oculoplastic specialist
in the management of Bell's Palsy?**
An oculoplastic specialist is involved in protecting the eye. Because the muscles around the eye are not functioning properly, the eyelids cannot close completely. This allows the eye to dry out—potentially leading to ulceration, infections and vision loss. This could also be very painful. Initially, protection of the eye is accomplished by aggressive eye lubrication and taping the eye shut at night. Sometimes the eye needs to be temporarily closed with a minor surgical technique. Most patients are not very agreeable to this. A more common method of allowing the eyelid to close better is with the use of a gold weight inserted surgically in the upper eyelid. This allows gravity to help close the eyelid with an attempted blink. Because the eyelid is not surgically closed, acceptance is much greater with this procedure. Maximal vision is maintained. I have been using gold weights for many years with excellent results. These weights are usually temporary. Once the palsy has resolved or the eye is no longer threatened, the weight can be removed with a simple surgical procedure. Once the palsy has resolved or stabilized, patients are still checked regularly.

Patients with chronic facial palsy can have further plastic surgery of the face and eyelids for functional and aesthetic improvement. Frequently, this is performed using an advanced reconstructive team approach.

CHAPTER EIGHT

EYELID GROWTHS-
ARE THEY BENIGN OR CANCEROUS?

Growths on the eyelid are very common. Probably the most common oculoplastic consultation I see is to evaluate a growth on the eyelid. They can be single or multiple and involve one or more of the eyelids. Multiple growths tend to be benign. Single growths raise more suspicion. Fortunately, benign eyelid growths tend to be more common, especially in the younger patient (Figures 12 & 13).

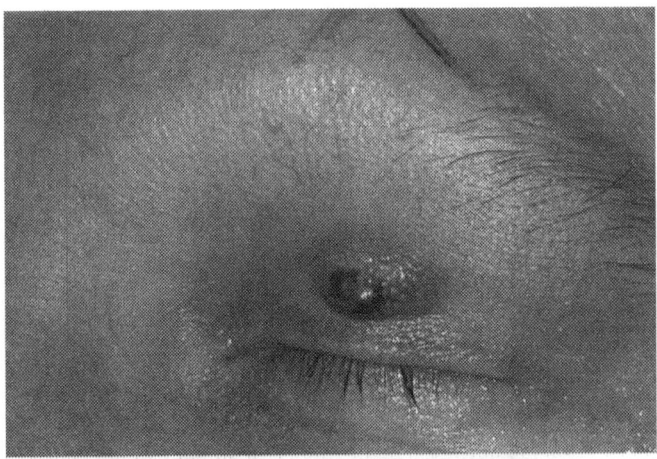

Fig. 12 This patient has a benign blood vessel growth called a hemangioma

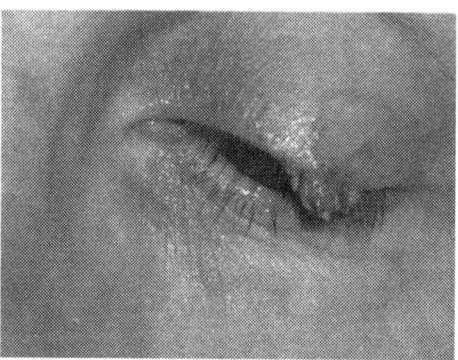

Fig. 13 This papillomatous growth
is benign and sometimes caused
by a virus

What should I do if I notice a growth on my eyelid?
It is best to have an ophthalmologist (MD) or oculoplastic specialist
evaluate any eyelid growth. These physicians can best examine your
eyelids under magnification to better define the problem. A complete
history is very important in deciding how to treat these lesions
(Figure 14). Some growths are treated with observation, antibiotics
or biopsy (see below). One of the most common infections in the
eyelid is a chalazion (Fig 14a). People often mistake a chalazion for
a "stye". Initial treatment is with warm compresses and antibiotics.

Some chalazions will eventually need to be surgically removed.

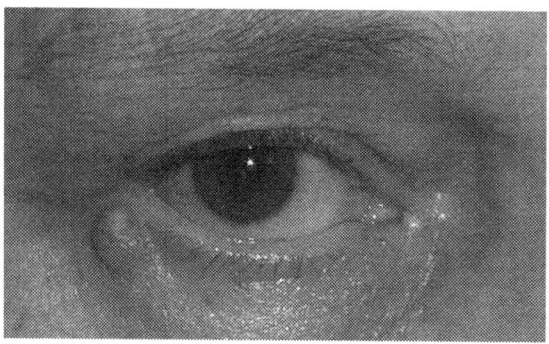

Fig 14. Sometimes it is necessary
to perform a biopsy to make the
diagnosis

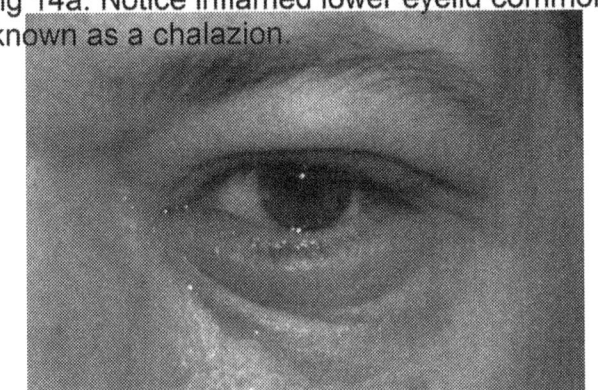
Fig 14a: Notice inflamed lower eyelid commonly known as a chalazion.

What historical information and physical findings are important for evaluation?

1. Your eye physician will want to know if any infection preceded the growth. Some eyelid infections will persist as cysts once treated.

2. The length of time that the growth has been present is important.

3. Is pain present? Does it hurt to touch the growth?

4. Has there been growth- and over what period of time? (Figures 15 & 15a)

5. Has the growth ever ulcerated and bled?

6. Did you or do you spend a lot of time in the sun?

7. Have you ever had any growths like this in the past?

8. Are your eyelashes missing?

9. Does the growth have irregular margins and irregular shapes? Remember that malignancies tend to destroy normal tissue

10. Are there any color changes?

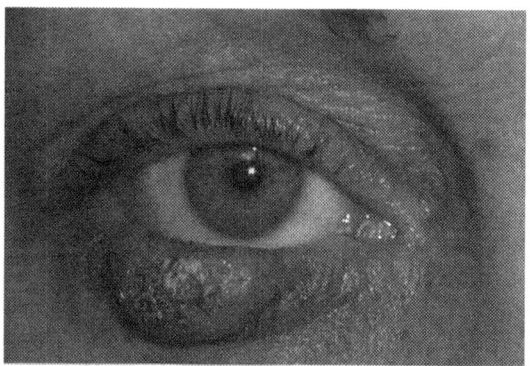

Fig 15. This growth grew rapidly
over a number of weeks and
turned out to be a
keratoacanthoma sometimes
confused as a malignant
process

Fig 15a: After many months, this growth
spontaneously heals. Note loss of
eyelashes

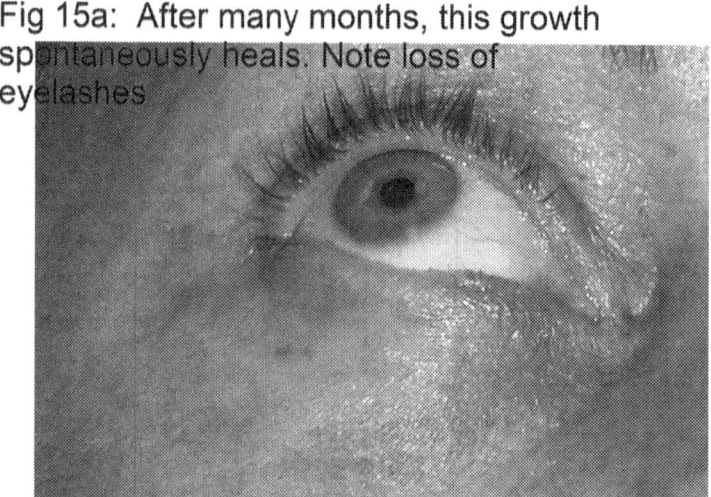

Based on the history and physical examination, if your eye physician is suspicious that the growth may be malignant, a biopsy will be suggested. In general benign growths have a uniform color with regular shapes and borders. Most pigmented growths are benign such as a **nevus (commonly called a mole).** Making sure a lid growth is not a malignancy is the main goal of the evaluation. Biopsies can be either incisional (removing a portion of the tumor) or excisional (removing the entire tumor). Some patients will frequently ask, "why not just remove the entire growth if you suspect it may be malignant"? The reason is that if the biopsy confirms malignancy, the surgical resection needs to be more extensive to insure complete removal. If it is benign, why remove unnecessary healthy tissue? In addition, there are a number of surgical options and techniques available that need to be discussed.

If a malignancy is determined by biopsy, what are my options?
Further surgery is definitely indicated. Almost all forms of eyelid skin cancer can be **cured** by **complete** removal. The most common form of eyelid skin cancer is a **basal cell carcinoma (Figure 16).** Basal cell carcinomas comprise more than 90% of malignant eyelid growths. These are caused by excessive exposure to sunlight and are usually seen after the age of sixty. I have, however, been seeing these cancers in younger patients in there forties and fifties. They tend to be more common in lighter skinned individuals with light skin and blue eyes. The second most common type of eyelid skin cancer is a **squamous cell carcinoma** (less than 5%). Squamous cell carcinoma is a more serious form because it can spread to distant sites and metastasize. A premalignant lesion **called actinic keratosis** occurs on sun damaged areas. Actinic keratosis can be a precursor to squamous cell carcinoma or a basal cell carcinoma. Actinic keratosis usually feels gritty to touch on the skin. Actinic keratosis needs to be treated. This is usually done by a dermatologist (doctor who specializes in the skin). Basal cell carcinomas tend only to spread locally. However, basal cell carcinomas if left untreated can spread

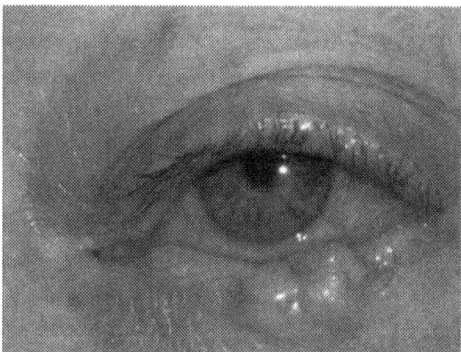

Fig 16. Basal Cell Carcinoma of
the lower eyelid, a malignant
skin cancer

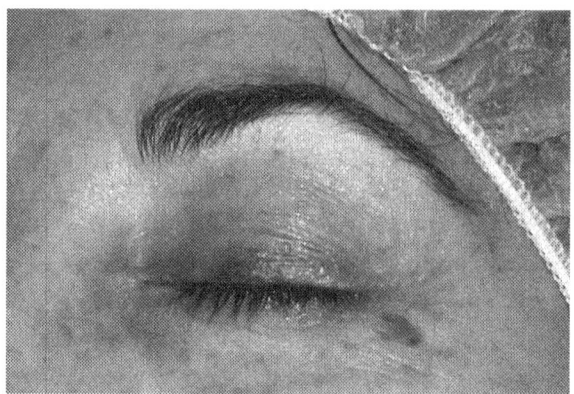

Fig 17. Pigmented growth of the
upper eyelid

behind the eye and to the brain. Another less commonly seen
malignant eyelid tumor is a **meibomian gland or sebaceous cell
carcinoma.** This can be a very dangerous malignancy resulting
in distant spread and death.   Meibomian gland carcinoma
often will masquerade as different eyelid growths.   A high
index of suspicion is necessary for making this diagnosis. A full
thickness eyelid biopsy (which involves all layers of the eyelid)
is the only way with special fat stains. Alerting the pathologist
(the doctor who examines the biopsy) to this possibility is very
important. I am also very suspicious of pigmented growths of

the eyelid (Figure 17). Because I am worried about a deadly cancer called **malignant melanoma**, I do not hesitate to biopsy pigmented lesions. Fortunately most pigmented growths are not melanomas. Remember that any skin growth may be pigmented.

After the biopsy returns as positive, I usually have an extensive discussion with my patients regarding their options. One thing is for certain. Further surgery with complete excision is now indicated and is the goal. The diagnosis will determine how much further tissue needs to be removed. In surgical lingo, this is known as "margin control".

The first option to consider is a technique called Moh's chemosurgery. This is performed by a specially trained dermatologist. The Moh's surgeon carefully removes the entire tumor trying to preserve as much normal tissue as possible (Figure 18). In conjunction with the Moh's surgeon, an oculoplastic surgeon will then do the eyelid reconstruction. That is, the plastic surgery to repair the defect created by the tumor removal.

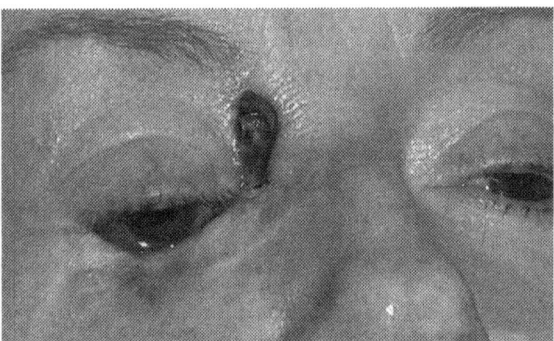

Fig 18. This patient had a basal cell carcinoma removed by the Moh's technique

The other method to consider is called frozen section controlled removal of the malignancy. This technique involves removing the main specimen and then taking pieces around the defect and examining to see if any tumor remains. Surgery continues until all tissue is free of tumor. Reconstruction proceeds as described for Moh's surgery.

The literature states that with Moh's surgery the cure rate is between 95%-98% for most basal cell carcinomas and between 95%-96% for excision with frozen section control.

It is the oculoplastic surgeon who is skilled in repairing all eyelid defects and restoring the eyelid back to a normal function and acceptable appearance. I always tell patients that there are three goals in malignant eyelid tumor surgery in this order. First, we need to get the entire tumor out to insure a low recurrence rate. Second, my job as an oculoplastic surgeon is to make the eyelid function again. It must be remembered that both the upper and lower eyelids serve a very important function in protecting the eye. And third, I use all my skills to make the eyelid appear as normal as possible. Sometimes with large defects this is not always possible. The final result can take up to six months before the eyelid reconstruction is fully healed.

Eyelid tumors can occur in children at any age and are handled in a similar manner. It is somewhat more difficult because removal usually necessitates a general anesthetic.

CHAPTER NINE

HOW DO I GET RID OF THESE WRINKLES?
(INCLUDING A DISCUSSION OF BOTOX, FILLERS, AND SKIN REJUVENATION)

Are all wrinkles the same?
I like to categorize wrinkles into two general types. There are
static wrinkles and there are **dynamic wrinkles**. Static wrinkles
are present with your facial muscles at rest. That is, you are not
smiling, talking or eating. Static wrinkles are present all the time
(Figure 19). Dynamic wrinkles, on the other hand, are present
when the facial muscles are active. Examples of dynamic wrinkles
include worsening of crow's feet when smiling or forehead lines
with eyebrow movement (Figure 20). This distinction needs to be
clearly understood because treatment depends on the type of wrinkle.
Both types are frequently addressed in an overall treatment plan.

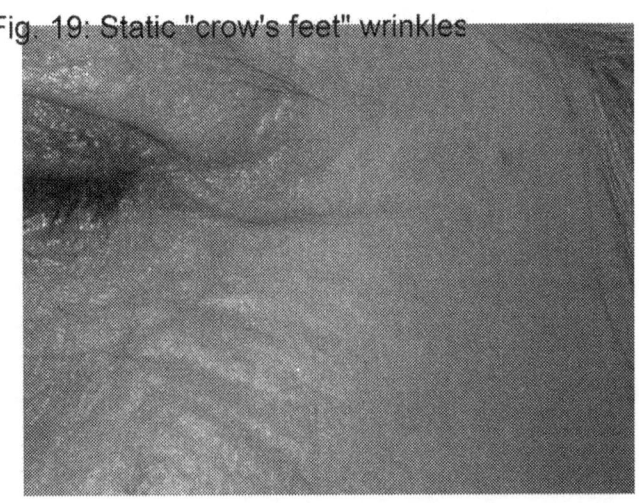

Fig. 19: Static "crow's feet" wrinkles

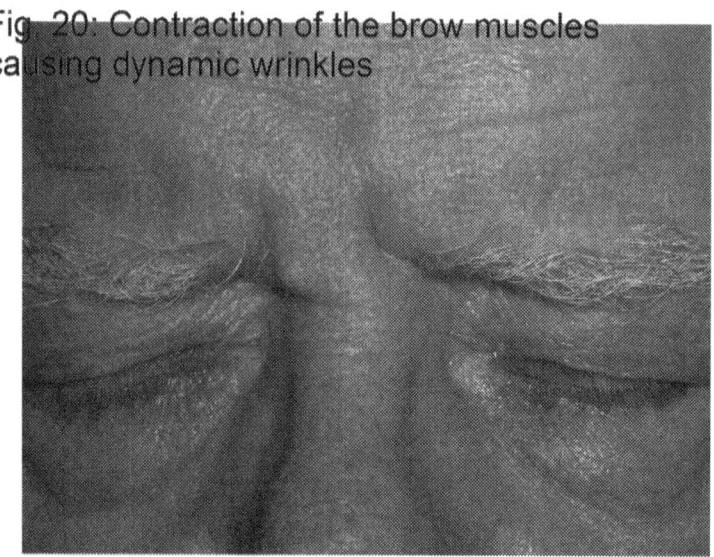

Fig. 20: Contraction of the brow muscles causing dynamic wrinkles

Why do wrinkles form?

I believe that the stimulus for wrinkle formation begins as soon as our facial muscles begin to work. Why they don't become noticeable for decades has to do with a number of factors. As we begin to age, the deeper skin tissue called collagen begins to disappear. This allows the skin to lose its' shape and thin out. The ability of the skin to keep its' fullness and elasticity diminishes. Coupled with the constant contraction of the facial muscles, creases begin to form. These eventually become wrinkles.

I believe that part of a person's ability to retain a youthful appearance has to do with heredity, their genes. However, I am also a firm believer that this can be modified in many ways. **The single most important external factor prematurely aging the skin is sun exposure.** It is often stated that 80% of your total lifetime sun exposure occurs before the age of 30, yet the effects are not seen until decades later. Unfortunately, it is very difficult to convey to young people the dangers of sun exposure in later life. I recommend to all my patients that they use sunscreens all year long with a block protection of at least 20. For women this should be easy to do because most facial moisturizers now contain sunblocks. These products are used everyday by most women. For men, this becomes more difficult. I personally use a moisturizing sunblock on my face all year long. I never sunbathe and I avoid prolonged sun exposure (even on the golf course!).

In addition, I believe that proper nutrition combined with a good exercise regimen can only enhance the anti-aging factors of the skin. Regular exercise increases blood flow to the skin, which clears out harmful chemicals that predispose to aging. Drinking plenty of water adds to the firmness of the skin. There is some evidence to believe that sleep patterns might contribute to premature wrinkling. There may be some theoretical advantage to sleeping on your back if you are comfortable doing this. I personally am not. I also recommend a daily vitamin with antioxidants. There is evidence to suggest that antioxidants are beneficial to general eye health as well.

What treatments are available?
The most important treatment is to minimize those factors that can accelerate aging of the skin. We discussed these in the previous question. For those patients that do desire treatment for their wrinkles, the first determination needs to made about what type of wrinkles are present—static or dynamic. Usually it is a combination of both.

Altering the skin surface usually treats static wrinkles. The techniques vary by modality used and the depth of penetration into the skin. These include:

1. Dermabrasion: an abrasive instrument is used to smooth the surface of the skin. This technique causes the most bleeding and is the least predictive.

2. Chemical peels: with this technique chemicals are used to remove the "bad" skin and new skin will replace it. Usually this new skin is of a better quality than the skin being removed. The strength of the chemical will determine the depth of penetration into the skin. These treatments are very effective.

3. Laser ablations: laser resurfacing was introduced about ten years ago. The CO2/Erbium laser is still the gold standard. However, the difficulty with CO2/Erbium laser resurfacing is the prolonged healing and downtime. This has led to a decrease in its use. Newer types of lasers called non-ablative lasers are being used. The problem that I see with these lasers is they are less effective than the CO2/Erbium laser. Results are not as impressive. The one big advantage is the significantly reduced downtime.

4. Fillers: fillers are substances that are injected under the surface of the skin. They are usually used as adjuvant treatment for persistent deeper furrows. We will talk more about this in the subsequent sections.

The best treatment for dynamic lines and wrinkles is botulinum toxin (Botox). Wrinkles usually result from muscle contraction and the aging changes of the skin.

My experience with most patients is that they have varying forms of both static and dynamic wrinkles. Usually treatment will consist of some combination of an ablative procedure (i.e. laser resurfacing, chemical peel), fillers and botulinun toxin. As mentioned above, non-ablative skin rejuvenation procedures have recently become popular because of decreased downtime allowing for a more rapid return to normal activities. Let's explore these in more detail.

Botulinum toxin (Botox) has been approved by the FDA for crossed eyes and eyelid spasms since 1989. It had been used investigationally since the early 1980's for these conditions. In 2002, botox was approved by the FDA for wrinkles between the eyebrows (glabella). Off label uses are commonly used for other wrinkles and frown lines (i.e. crows' feet and lip lines). Botox blocks the ability of muscles to contract by blocking the release of a chemical necessary for contraction. With less movement, the skin gradually begins to smooth out. Sometimes an anesthetic cream can be used on the skin 30 minutes to one hour before treatment. In my experience, I rarely use any anesthetic in most patients. Ice packs frequently work nicely to help with any discomfort from the injections. The effect is usually seen in 2-3 weeks but can occur in the first week after treatment. The effect is temporary, lasting anywhere from 3-6 months. A number of different types of botulinum toxins are produced commercially, type A (Botox and Dysport) and type B (Myobloc).

Included in **Table 1** is my consent form that discusses botox treatment and possible side effects.

TABLE 1

PATIENT CONSENT FOR ADMINISTRATION OF BOTOX

- **I request that Ronald Kristan, MD administer botulinum toxin to me for either medical or cosmetic purposes. Botox, as of this writing, is not approved for headache treatment.**

- **If the drug is being administered for medical purposes, such as involuntary muscle spasms, blepharospasm, hemi facial spasm, muscle twitch or tick, etc., I hereby acknowledge that I understand that there may be alternative treatments for this condition. These include, but are not limited to, medical therapy involving the administration of oral medicines, muscle stripping or other operations, removal of motor nerves, or procedures to release pressure on the involved nerves.**

- **I acknowledge that I understand that Botox A includes human albumin. Human albumin is a protein, similar to the white of an egg, which is derived from human blood products. Based on effective donor screening and product manufacturing processes, it carries an extremely remote risk for transmission of viral diseases. A theoretical risk for transmission of Creutzfeldt-Jacob disease (CJD) also is considered extremely remote. No cases of transmission** of viral diseases or CJD have ever been identified for albumin. While it is not believed that there has been any transmission of disease from Botox A, I understand that this is very unlikely but possible.

- I accept the risk of the remote possibility of acquiring an infection from Botox administration and accept the risk of unknown future complications from Botox use. I understand that botulinum B can also be used for my condition and does not contain albumin.

- Botulinum toxin usually works well in 95% of patients. There is a 5% chance that it will not have an adequate effect. It is not always possible to predict the effect. It may work too well or not well enough. Some of the side effects may include temporary droopiness of one or both eyelids, double vision, redness and bruising at the injection sites, headache, respiratory infections, flu symptoms, nausea and facial pain.

- Permanent muscle weakness is very unlikely. Antibodies to Botox may reduce the effectiveness of subsequent treatments. The development of antibodies has not been well studied.

- I understand that the effects of botulinum toxin use with pregnancy or breast-feeding are not known. I should not take Botox if the possibility of pregnancy or nursing exists.

- I have informed Dr. Kristan of any neuromuscular disorders that I have such as ALS, myasthenia gravis, or Lambert-Eaton syndrome.

- In summary, the risks, consequences, benefits and alternatives of treatment, including no treatment, have been explained to me. All my questions have been answered.

Botox treatment involves making a number of injections with a very tiny needle to relax the desired muscles. The treatment is quick and minimally invasive. Patients return back to their regular routine immediately. Most of my patients do not complain of significant discomfort. I still believe the expressions of the face should be maintained. I believe the results should be subtle with a refreshed look.

Dermal fillers have recently undergone resurgence in interest and usage. Fillers allow facial features to achieve more fullness. Fullness defines a more youthful look. Fillers restore volume to the skin and allow for the correction of moderate to severe facial wrinkles and folds. One such fold, the **nasolabial fold** of the lower face is probably the most common area treated with fillers.

Dermal fillers can be classified into two broad categories:

Degradable (effects lessen with time)

1. **Collagen (usually last less than 3 months)**

    a. bovine: these include **zyderm (1and 2)** and **zyplast (comparable to zyderm plus lidocaine, a local anesthetic).** Zyderm can be used to treat fine lines, wrinkles and shallow scars. Zyderm is indicated for thin-skin areas. Zyplast is more viscous and can be used to treat more significant lines, wrinkles and scars. It can also be used in thicker skinned areas.

    b. porcine

    c. bioengineered human: The more recently approved **cosmoderm** and **cosmoplast** behave similarly to zyderm and zyplast in their indications and usage.

2. **Hyaluronic Acid: Hyaluronic acid is a naturally occurring substance in the body-often referred to as "sugar gel". The most popular hyaluronic acids are restylane, perlane(a thicker restylane) and hylaform. Hylaform is avian derived whereas restylane and perlane are non animal derived. Hylaform tends to last about three months whereas**

restylane tends to last four to six months. The hyaluronic acid fillers have been associated with minimal allergic reactions. They absorb water and hence last longer than collagen fillers. However, they tend not to flow as easily as collagen. (Figure 20a)

Pre injection of   Post injection of
restylane   restylane

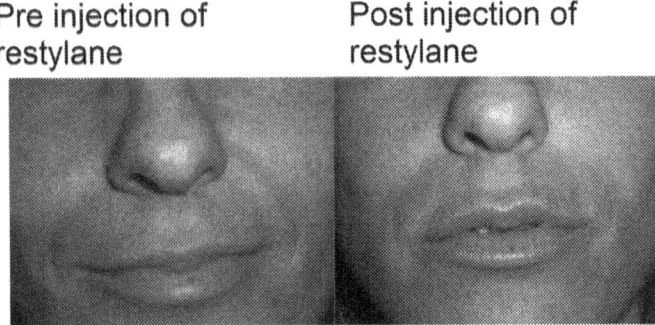

3. **Autologous Fat: this is fat taken from one part of your own body to be used as a filler. This is probably the safest, but the effects are variable. Complications include bleeding, infection, stroke and cyst formation.**

Let's talk in more detail about **restylane**. Because restylane is a non-animal based product, the risks of animal-based disease transmission or allergic reactions are minimal. Unlike collagen (except for cosmoderm and cosmoplast), restylane requires no pre-allergy testing. As with any invasive procedure, any medications that can increase bleeding (such as aspirin and Vitamin E) should be stopped before the injections. Typically, the injections will require the use of a local anesthetic (that is novocain). Usually bruising, redness, and swelling occur after the treatment. This will resolve within the first week. Restylane has been primarily used on the lower face. Recently, however, treatments for lower eyelids and brow are being investigated with encouraging results. Based on these early results, I feel that eyelid and brow uses for restylane will continue to expand. **Perlane** is a thicker form of restylane and may be used for more pronounced filling. Perlane may also last longer than restylane.

Non-Biodegradable Synthetic fillers that are currently available in the United States can be classified as **injectables (Artecoll and Silicone) and implants (GORE-TEX and Ultrasoft).** These fillers tend to be used for longer-term correction of skin and soft tissue defects. They tend to be associated with more problems. I have very little experience with these non-biodegradable synthetic fillers.

It must be remembered that the use of dermal fillers is really an art-like sculpting. Everyone needs to be individualized and touch-ups may be necessary.

SKIN REJUVENATION

The previous section dealt with techniques that are effective for wrinkle and gravitational effects of aging. This section will deal with methods of improving the **quality** of the skin caused by aging, sun exposure (photo damage) and gravitational changes. These techniques can be used to treat sun spots and pigmentary changes of the skin. They can also help with fine wrinkle removal.

I break these techniques into **ablative skin resurfacing, nonablative skin resurfacing, chemical dermabrasion, and cosmeceuticals.**

Ablative Skin Resurfacing:
Ablative skin resurfacing actually removes the superficial layers of the skin down to the dermis (layer right under the surface). As a result the skin appears as if it was "burned". I tell patients the immediate post operative result will look like a bad sunburn.

The two main lasers used for ablative treatments are the **CO2 Laser and the Erbium Laser.** In my opinion, the CO2 laser is more effective in treating fine wrinkles and photo damaged tissue. However, the CO2 laser causes far more tissue reaction requiring more intensive post-operative care. Patients need to be seen frequently in the office in the first two weeks after surgery and can't be very social because of facial crusting and pain. The skin oozes for about a week and remains red for many weeks to months (and rarely years). Infection is always a possibility as are cold sores (herpes simplex). Irregular scarring and increased skin pigmentation are potential complications.

There is a lot of care required for an optimal result. The Erbium laser is associated with less reaction that the CO2 laser-but I feel the results are not as good. Many patients will choose the Erbium option because of less down time and post operative care. I find that less patients choose these options because of the required after care.

A newer type of ablative resurfacing is called **fractal resurfacing**. With this technique a small area of skin is treated while the adjacent area is left intact. This pattern is repeated throughout the entire treatment zone. The concept here is that the uninjured skin provides for more rapid healing of the treated area at the same time the skin is rejuvenated.

Nonablative Skin Resurfacing:
Because of the significant post-operative care of ablative therapy, nonablative techniques have become more popular. I believe that at this writing, the nonablative therapies available are not as effective as the ablative lasers. However, they do offer patients an option for skin rejuvenation that has virtually no downtime and much less post-operative care. These devices do not remove the superficial layers of the skin. They penetrate through skin to the deeper layers where they work to stimulate collagen development. Collagen in the deeper skin is what keeps the skin firm and plump-characteristics of youthful skin. This is a rapidly changing field of skin rejuvenation and I feel it will continue to do so. Some of the available technologies at this writing include:

  i. Radiofrequency Devices: Radiofrequency has been used for many years as a surgical tool to cut tissue. Recently it has been adapted as a noninvasive device for delivery of energy to the dermis to stimulate collagen growth. Included in this group are the Thermage system, and the Syneron elos system.

ii. Intense Pulse Light (IPL): IPL targets wrinkle removal, pigment removal and vascular (i.e. rosacea) areas. Advantages of IPL include speed, little downtime, and minimal discomfort. Recently the use of a photochemical called leuvlan (alpha-aminolevulenic acid) appears to improve the photorejuvenation efficiency. This technique is also thought to stimulate collagen production. The method of improving pigmentary/vascular problems relates to specific wavelength targeting of these areas. Complications include redness, bruising and blistering.

iii. Cool Touch Rejuvenation Lasers: these lasers involve cooling the skin surface prior to laser treatment. Multiple applications are frequently necessary.

iv. Gentle Waves: this is newest form of non-ablative skin rejuvenation involving light emitting diode (LED) technology. LED energy stimulates cellular activity such as wound healing. Exposure to LED at a specific wavelength is thought to activate cells to produce collagen-helping to maintain healthy looking skin. This system is usually integrated with a complete skin care program designed to enhance and maintain the results of treatment. Advantages to this technique include no known side effects, downtime or pain. The treatment is fast and convenient and treats the entire face all at once. The downside is that multiple treatments are needed (8-9) for the full effect to be seen. Maintenance treatments are necessary.

Dermabrasion:

I break dermabrasion down into two categories. One, chemicals are applied to the skin, kept on for a certain period of time, and then wiped off. This technique is commonly referred to as "a peel". Superficial peels are done with trichloroacetic acid and deeper peels with phenols. The effect of the peel depends on the strength of the chemical applied, how long it stays on the skin, and skin thickness/ type. The second type of dermabrasion is done mechanically with a surgical instrument that actually removes the outer layer of skin-almost like sandpaper. Some dermabrasion techniques can actually cause the skin to bleed whereas **microdermabrasion** involves only superficial treatment. It is the subsequent healing that creates the rejuvenation of the skin with both techniques. My experience is that the end point for these techniques is harder than for laser rejuvenation.

Cosmeceuticals:
Skin care helps to slow down the process of aging. Cosmeceuticals involves the use of skin care products that have a basis in biological science. Cosmeceuticals also enhance the benefits of eyelid surgery.

As I have mentioned elsewhere in this book, I believe that sun exposure is the single most important external factor involved in aging of the skin. **Therefore, the most important skin protection cosmeceutical is a sun block**. This protects against both UV B and UV A radiation. It is UV A radiation that is thought to be responsible for skin cancer. Sun blocks like zinc oxide protect the skin better than sun screens. Sun screens are absorbed by the skin and have less UV A protection than sun blocks.

Antioxidants are probably the next most important cosmeceutical. They block damage from free radical formation at the cellular level, protecting against photo aging. Included in this category are topical vitamin C, E and zinc. Alpha-lipoic acid is part of the enzyme complex responsible for oxidative metabolism. It can be used topically and orally. Another antioxidant, pycnogenol, is thought to work together with vitamins C and E.

Synthetic drugs called **retinoids** have been shown to improve fine lines, pigmented spots and the general texture of the skin. These include Retin-A and Renova, Tazorac and Azelex. **Alpha-hydroxy acids** are often used as a complement to retinoids. These are naturally occurring acids and are less irritating than retinoids.

Cosmeceuticals are a growing field in the skin care industry. As better science defines the aging process, more options will continue to be developed.

CHAPTER TEN

I HAVE THYROID DISEASE-
CAN IT AFFECT MY EYES?

Thyroid Disease can affect the body in many ways. Basically, either you produce too much thyroid hormone or not enough. Thyroid hormone is critical in maintaining many of the metabolic functions of the body, like temperature and activity levels. Usually, if you are making too much thyroid hormone, you are always warm and very hyperactive. Underproduction of thyroid hormone results in feeling cold, tired and sluggish. A very common type of hyperactive thyroid is called **Graves Disease.** Eye and eyelid findings are often seen in patients with Graves Disease (Figure 21). All patients diagnosed with thyroid abnormalities must have a thorough eye evaluation. Graves disease is five times more likely to affect women than men. Genetic factors appear to have a role in the development of thyroid associated orbitopathy, with 20%-60% of those affected reported to have a familial history of thyroid disease.

Fig 21: This patient has lid retraction on the right side and ptosis of the left upper lid

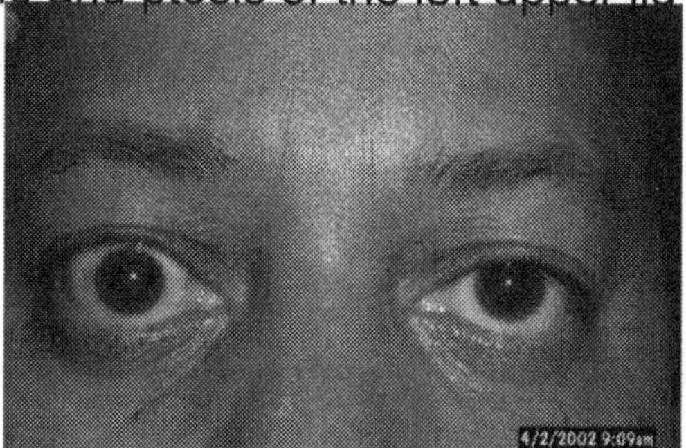

Environmental factors are also important in Graves disease. Cigarette smoking is capable of aggravating and prolonging thyroid-associated orbital inflammation. Approximately 20% of patients presenting with Graves disease will have some clinical evidence of Graves eye disease.

What are the eye/eyelid findings seen with thyroid disease?
Dry, scratchy eyes are frequently present. This can be treated with topical lubrication both during the day and at bedtime. Eyelid findings include eyelid retraction, especially of the upper lid (Figure 22). With this sign, the upper eyelid is at a higher position than normal, causing the eye to appear too wide open. Another common finding is that the eyes can "bulge" forward. This, coupled with eyelid retraction, can give the very characteristic appearance of very prominent eyes. Usually this results in irritation and congestion of the eye. Treatment with tear drops and anti-inflammatory drops is frequently prescribed. If dryness and ulceration occur, infection is possible. These can be serious requiring urgent treatment. Sleeping with your head elevated often helps with the congestion.

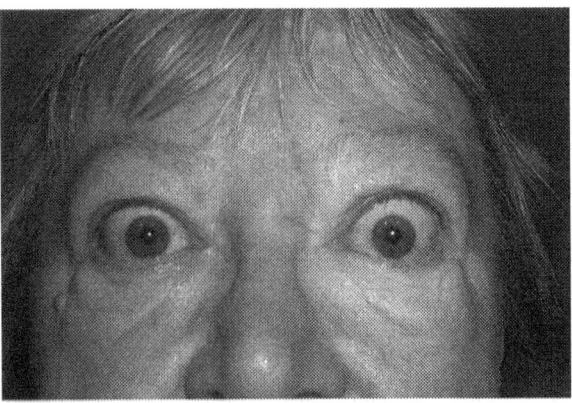

Fig 22. Upper and lower eyelid retraction. Eyes appear to bulge

Other less common signs include double vision caused by involvement of the muscles that move the eye.

A more serious situation can occur if there is compression of the optic nerve. This results from congestion and swelling of the eye muscles. This can cause permanent loss of vision. Optic nerve compression is considered a medical emergency. The severity and duration of the disease are unpredictable.

Radioactive iodine treatment for hyperactive thyroid has been reported to exacerbate preexisting orbital signs and symptoms. This is, however, somewhat controversial. In patients with severe optic nerve disease, radioactive iodine should be avoided or delayed.

In the pediatric population, eye findings are less common.

Besides the regular eye exam, what other testing is done?
The most common blood test to identify thyroid abnormalities is the thyroid-stimulating hormone or TSH. A T3 and T4 level is also standard. In addition levels of thyroid autoantibodies frequently helps make the diagnosis.

Because vision loss from optic nerve compression is so important, I usually obtain a visual field test (a measurement of the optic nerve function), color testing (sensitive measurement of the optic nerve), and an MRI scan of the orbits. The MRI scan images the optic nerve and muscles better than a CT scan. Some authorities, however, feel CT scanning is the gold standard for the diagnosis and treatment of Graves because of better bone resolution. Either scan allows direct visualization of the optic nerve and can be used as a reference for future scans if the clinical situation warrants it.

What treatments are available for thyroid eye disease?
Fortunately, most patients with thyroid eye disease require symptomatic treatment only. That is tear supplements and lubricating drops. I recommend that patients consider sleeping with their heads elevated if possible. This minimizes the orbital congestion that occurs at night. Limiting salt intake, and good wrap around sunglasses are also a must. Most thyroid eye disease

will run a course of a couple of years. The goals of therapy are to prevent ulceration, infection and loss of vision. Patient comfort is also a priority.

Once the thyroid disease is stable, eyelid surgery for lid retraction and strabismus surgery for diplopia (double vision) can be entertained.

If optic nerve compression is present, treatment must be urgent. Cortisone by mouth, radiation and surgery are all options. Surgery consists of decompressing the tissues around the eye to relieve any pressure on the eye.

As mentioned above, all patients with thyroid disease need to have regular visits with the oculoplastic specialist. This will depend on the severity of the disease and the eye findings. I feel very strongly about constant communication with patients during this difficult time. Support for patients is vital for their care.

Remember that improvement in the eye disease does not necessarily follow successful treatment of the systemic disease.

Can thyroid eye findings be present without obvious evidence of thyroid disease?
This concept gets a little tricky. The answer is yes. It is generally well accepted that some patients present to the eye doctor with eye/eyelid findings suggestive of thyroid disease. These were discussed above. However, when these patients are checked for thyroid disease by the standard testing, their thyroid values are normal. Also, they have no symptoms of systemic thyroid disease on routine testing.

I will usually recommend to these patients that they consult with an endocrinologist, a medical doctor who specializes in thyroid disease. An endocrinologist can perform more sophisticated blood studies that can confirm the presence of thyroid disease. Even if the studies are negative, patients with eye findings are categorized as having **euthyroid eye disease.** I follow these patients carefully with their endocrinologist and treat any eye disease as described above.

CHAPTER ELEVEN

WHY DO MY EYES BLINK ALL THE TIME?

My eyes seem to blink all the time—is something wrong?
Blinking can be caused by many factors. Something may be wrong. When I first went into practice, I saw a number of patients who had consulted with me for this problem. Most had been to a handful of doctors only to be told there was nothing wrong. Many patients went undiagnosed for years. Most of these patients, however, suffered from a condition called benign essential blepharospasm or BEB for short. This prompted me to conduct a study related to all the factors involved in diagnosing this condition. I was surprised to discover how little the medical community knew about BEB. This was the start of an interest of mine that has continued to this day, that is, taking care of patients with benign essential blepharospasm. Conditions related to over activity of the facial muscles include: **facial tics, orbicularis spasms (myokymia), hemifacial spasm and benign essential blepharospasm.**

Facial tics and orbicularis myokymia are usually self limited. Orbicularis myokymia can last anywhere from a few weeks to a few months and is almost always benign. It begins spontaneously and usually stops spontaneously. If it persists constantly for a number of months I will recommend a neurological workup. I have used botulinum toxin for this condition if a complete neurological evaluation is negative. Facial tics are often stress related. This chapter will primarily discuss BEB and hemifacial spasm.

What is Benign Essential Blepharospasm (BEB)?
BEB is an involuntary forceful closure of the eyelids in the absence of eyelid, ocular or central nervous system disease (Figure 23).

Figure 23. This patient has benign essential blepharospasm and is functionally blind

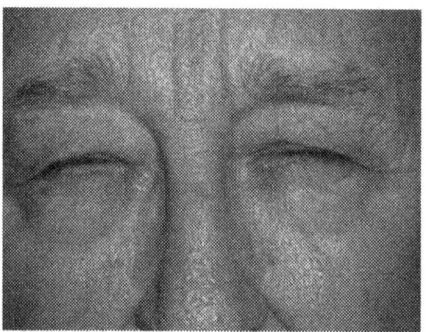

Much research is being done, but a true cause has not been found. The cause, however, appears to be multifactorial. A genetic predisposition with an environmental trigger seems to be supported by animal models.

BEB is usually a chronic disorder. This form of blepharospasm is considered "benign" because there is no known medical reason such as a tumor or degenerative disease like multiple sclerosis. I have not seen a patient have a spontaneous remission. This has been reported in a small percentage of BEB usually within the first five years of diagnosis.

The incidence in women is about two times greater than in men. The usual age of onset is between 40 and 50. Interestingly, dry eye may a trigger in BEB. Dry eye also appears to be common in postmenopausal women, which is a common age for the onset of BEB. In a recent survey, approximately 40% of patients stated that their occupation was doing some sort of clerical work. It may be that the eye strain associated with clerical work can cause an abnormal blink reflex, initiating blepharospasms. The primary problem is in the part of the brain that controls eyelid closure. Positron emission tomography (PET) scans show increased activity in the pons, basal ganglia, thalamus and cerebellum. Approximately 30% of patients report a positive family history. Complex genetic mechanisms are beginning to emerge through genetic research. BEB is not fatal. Some patients have had previous head or eye trauma.

What are the symptoms of BEB?
Blepharospasm often begins with increased frequency of blinking. Remember that the normal blink rate is about 20 times per minute. Patients with BEB have varying degrees of eyelid closure. Minimal spasms to complete closure can be seen. This makes patients functionally blind and interferes with all aspects of their lives. Just imagine driving and your eyelids go into a spasm and cause your eyes to close. This could be a very dangerous situation. Patients with BEB are usually healthy with no other medical problems. Older patients with BEB can have associated problems such as high blood pressure and diabetes. Blepharospasm patients have higher light sensitivity than normal people.

Eyelid spasms usually occur spontaneously, but can be aggravated by bright lights or irritants to the eyes such as wind or smoke. Patients might initially describe eye irritation, burning or eye discomfort. Subsequently, patients complain of more severe blinking and light sensitivity (**photophobia**). Recent studies have shown that photophobia is very common and that light is an important trigger for blepharospasm. Sometimes BEB can be accompanied by other spasms of the lower face and neck (also called **Meige syndrome**).

Some patients present with spasms involving only half of their face. This is called **hemifacial spasm.**

All patients with BEB and the variants described above require a complete medical and neurological work-up (including MRI scanning) prior to initiating any treatments. Newer imaging studies, like the PET scan (positron emission tomography), are beginning to elucidate abnormalities in specific nerve pathways in the brain (more specifically the putamen in the basal ganglion). There are no specific blood tests or scans for diagnosing BEB and its' related disorders.

What treatments are available for BEB?
A small percentage of patients can go into remission (less than 5%). Once established, however, there is a very small chance of remission. There is no know cure for BEB. Treatments are aimed at relieving symptoms. Botulinum toxin injection is the main treatment option for BEB. It has been used since the early 1980's for this condition. Botulinum toxin has been shown to be highly effective and safe. Side effects are minimal. (**see Table 1 Chapter Nine for list of side effects**). The only disadvantage is that the injections only last 3-6 months. There are eight know types (serotypes) of the toxin. These are described as A-G. The most common types used clinically are A and B. Botulinum toxin A is know as BOTOX in the United States and DYSPORT in Europe. The only form of botulinum B at this time is MYOBLOC. Myobloc is approved by the FDA for torticollis (neck spasms) but not yet for blepharospasm or hemifacial spasm. Myobloc can be used as an off label use, however, for blepharospasm. Only a small percentage (1%) of patients do not respond to botulinum treatment from the onset.

A number of medications have been tried as treatment for these conditions. The drugs that have had the most success are the GABA analogs. GABA is a chemical that works in the brain to enhance drowsiness and muscle relaxation. Anticholinergic agents block acetylcholine, the transmitter between the nerve and the muscle. These drugs can impair memory, cause drowsiness, blurred vision, constipation and urinary retention problems. Valium-like drugs, antihistamines, antiepileptic drugs have all been used. My experience is that because these drugs have a lot of side effects, their use is somewhat limited.

Another injectable medication, doxorubicin, has been used on a limited basis. Skin side effects have been an issue with this drug. Oral medications in my experience have been disappointing in the treatment of BEB.

Surgical treatments are performed less frequently now with the use of botulinum. Techniques included removal of 90% of the muscles around the eye and eyebrow, known as a myectomy. This was an effective treatment, however the surgery was complicated, risky, and had a long post-op recovery period. Most surgical procedures that are performed today are used as an adjunct to botulinum (known as a limited myectomy) or when botulinum therapy is no longer effective. This may include changing doses caused by a shift in muscle handling of the toxin or antibody formation due to previous toxin treatment. This is why it is important to extend out the treatment period as long as possible and give the lowest possible dose. Fortunately, the newer lower-protein BOTOX seems to associated with a lower risk of antibody formation. Modified blepharoplasties and ptosis surgery are standard operations at this time.

Patients with hemifacial spasm that are found to have vascular compression may benefit by decompression surgery performed by a neurosurgeon. This involves relieving the pressure caused by a small blood vessel on the seventh nerve as it exits the brain.

Various types of eyeglass tints (such as FL-41) may improve light sensitivity in these patients. Investigational treatments at this writing include liposome encapsulated chemomyectomy using doxorubicin. Other treatments that have been tried include acupuncture, hypnosis, bio-feedback and nutritional therapy. A recently conducted study using super blue-green algae in the treatment of blepharospasm has been completed. Overall there was no evidence of improvement in botox treatments when combined with super blue-green algae. There may be a slight benefit in patients younger than 60, however. You can certainly try super blue-green algae for a few months and if you notice no real response, then I would advise discontinuing it.

What other conditions can cause eyelid blinking or spasms?
1. **Dry Eyes: particular attention is paid to the tear film**. The tear film is composed of layers, just like a sandwich. There is a fatty (lipid) outer layer, a watery (aqueous) middle layer, and an inner mucous layer. Any disruption in the

sandwich can produce dry eyes and blepharospasm. The diagnosis of dry eyes needs to be established. Treatment with topical lubrication and punctal plugs can be tried. Restasis is a newer drop that is actually thought to increase the production of tears. The problem with restasis is that about 25% of patients cannot tolerate it because of increased irritation and sensitivity.

2. **Allergic Conjunctivitis**

3. **Eyelid inflammation: Rosacea/ blepharitis**

4. **Eyelid abnormalities such as misdirected eyelashes**

5. **Central Nervous System disease, brain tumors or seizure disorders**

6. **Uncorrected or incorrect eyeglass prescription**

7. **Psychogenic**

8. **Habit Tic**

9. **Tourette syndrome**

These conditions cause what we describe as **secondary blepharospasm.**

So as you can see, patients who present with eyelid spasms undergo an extensive work-up. A comprehensive ophthalmic and neurological evaluation is performed on every patient before the diagnosis of BEB is made.

What is Apraxia of Lid Opening?

Apraxia of eyelid opening is associated with BEB. These patients have difficulty opening their eyelids even after treatment with BOTOX. Although the eyelid spasms have been reduced, these patients appear to be failures or have minimal improvement.

In patients with apraxia of lid opening, involuntary lid closure results despite adequate botulinum treatment of the eyelid and brow muscles. The eyelids seem to droop close without obvious spasm, yet the levator muscle appears to be normal. Treatment includes myectomy (removal of orbicularis muscle) and ptosis repair (tightening of the levator muscle). Usually the brow muscles need to be used to elevate the eyelids in a procedure known as a frontalis suspension. A sling is used to attach the eyelid to the brow. Patients then lift their eyelids with the sling connected to the brow. There are many materials now being used as slings-from synthetic to donor material to autologous (patients' own tissue).

Does blepharospasm interfere with cataract surgery?
The biggest problem would be if you had any uncontrollable spasms during surgery. I always recommend paralyzing the muscles with local anesthetic just to ensure safety during the operation. Also spasms after surgery could cause tension on the incision. I try to recommend cataract surgery when the spasms are relatively controlled-usually one month after botox injections.

Patients with BEB and its related disorders should contact the **Benign Essential Blepharospasm Foundation** for further information. This organization has a wealth of information on these conditions. Newsletter, local support groups, meeting locations and ongoing research are some of the many resources available. Their web site is **www.blepharospasm.org**

CHAPTER TWELVE

Management of Eyelid Trauma

Eyelid trauma can result from many causes and result in many different types of injuries. Any time there is eye/eyelid trauma, the first plan of action is to make sure there has not been any damage to the eyeball. This is the first priority. Sometimes it is necessary to go to the operating room to rule out an eye injury. Once this has been done then the eyelids and surrounding areas can be evaluated.

Unfortunately, I have seen a significant amount of trauma in my career. Injuries ranging from dog bites to fishing hook injuries to fist fights. If you think that the eye can be injured during an activity-it probably has been. You always need to use common sense and carefully protect the eye and eyelid structures with safety glasses at all times. Participation in sports frequently produces periocular trauma.

Repair of eyelid trauma involves very careful assessment of the damage, loss of tissue and control of bleeding. Sometimes the tear duct drainage system is involved. Secondary procedures may be necessary. Most of the time CT scans or MRI scans are done prior to treatment. Trauma surgery requires a detailed knowledge of eyelid anatomy and function. Basic eyelid reconstruction techniques are followed to insure the best function and cosmetic appearance. This is where my training as an eyelid plastic surgeon is frequently challenged.

It is beyond the scope of this book to review all the myriad of surgical techniques of eyelid repair. My purpose with this short chapter was just to make you aware of another area that eyelid plastic surgeons often deal with.

CHAPTER THIRTEEN

EYE HEALTH, EXERCISE AND ALTERNATIVE TREATMENTS INCLUDING VITAMINS AND NUTRITION

We are constantly bombarded with information in the newspapers, magazines, TV and radio regarding alternative forms of treatment and health management. Sometimes it is difficult to sift through all this material. There always seems to a "vitamin of the month" or "magnet treatment" for a particular disorder or a new "herb' to treat cancer. Even as a physician, knowing what may be helpful to my patients is often frustrating to me.

Being trained as a scientist and with Western medical concepts, I still believe that any claim of medical effectiveness be backed up by solid studies. I have a very open mind with respect to alternative treatments. I believe that anything you can do to maintain your overall general health has to be good for the eyes. Over my almost twenty years in practice, I have developed what I call **Dr. Kristan's Common Sense Rules for a Healthy Life Style.** These are based on my interpretation of what is in the medical literature and observations with my patients. I believe that each one of us needs to control the risk factors.

Dr. Kristan's TEN COMMON SENSE RULES for a HEALTHY LIFE STYLE

1. Maintain proper weight: I believe that being overweight is the single most harmful thing that you can do to your body. Being overweight puts stresses on your heart, increases your blood pressure, makes you more prone to diabetes and increases your risk of stroke. I believe that people become over weight because of a lack of understanding of nutrition, little to no exercise and a lack of will power. Nearly two thirds of US adults are overweight. I will discuss weight issues in more detail later in this chapter.

2. Understand proper nutrition: I believe that most people do not understand the difference between carbohydrates, proteins and fat. I do not believe that any of the fad diets make sense. I have always felt that a proper combination of carbohydrates, protein and fat makes the most sense. I personally eat about 35% carbohydrates, 40% protein and 25% fat. I think that everyone needs to discover what combination works for him or her—combined with adequate exercise.

3. Exercise, exercise, and exercise! I can't stress this enough. I believe that the key to maintaining the proper weight is with exercise and good nutrition. Exercise increases the blood flow to the whole body. We know that that eye has a very high blood flow. This is required for good eye health. Anything that increases the blood flow to the eye has to be good for health maintenance. We also know that some forms of glaucoma may be related to decreased blood flow to the eye. Recently, some researchers have shown that aerobic exercise and strength training can reduce the intraocular pressure in both healthy and glaucoma patients. Some studies suggest a lowering effect of 10% to 20%. Exercise also helps to maintain normal blood pressure. My recommendation is at least 30 minutes of exercise/strength training three to four times a week. The

level of activity obviously needs to be dictated by physical health. Exercise benefits not only physical health buy also mental health.

4. Maintain normal blood pressure and have your blood sugars checked regularly: High blood pressure can lead to heart disease, kidney disease and stroke. In addition, high blood pressure can cause hemorrhaging in the eye that can lead to permanent visual loss.

    Diabetes can cause many problems throughout the body including the kidney, nervous system and the eye. If you have diabetes, keep in the best control you can. Keeping the HbA1C under 7 has been shown to decrease the incidence of complications.

5. STOP SMOKING: Smoking is a risk factor for a number of ocular diseases, including cataract and age-related macular degeneration. It is well known that smoking can affect the immune (the body's defense) system. As discussed in a previous chapter, thyroid disease can seriously affect the eyes. Smoking has definitely been shown to worsen the eye problems associated with thyroid disease. Smoking can also change the tear film in patients with dry eyes resulting in exacerbation of symptoms. Smoking definitely disturbs the circulatory system and may contribute to retinal vascular disease and "strokes" within the eye. I also feel that smoking contributes to premature aging of the skin, accelerating droopy upper and lower eyelids. These risks are on top of the well-known smoking risks of heart and lung disease, as well as generalized strokes. Over 400,000 people die each year from smoking related illnesses. Smokers are twice as likely to develop heart attacks as nonsmokers. Remember that it is never too late to stop smoking since your risk of heart disease definitely goes down after stopping. I have even seen statistics that state a former smoker's risk of heart disease comes close to a nonsmoker after 15 years.

6. Maintain DISCIPLINE: The most difficult task we have is sticking to our healthy plan. It is too easy to stray away from. Holidays, parties, good tasting (fatty) food—it is all around us. One needs to develop the will power to resist. In addition, I have an exercise routine that I do every week. I exercise Monday, Wednesday, Saturday and Sunday every week at the same time. Everyone in my family knows it and it is my time. I think about it like taking a shower every morning. It is just something I always do. Treat exercise just like something you must do regularly. If I can do it with my busy schedule as a physician, you can too.

7. Think POSITIVELY: I am a firm believer that people who have a positive attitude perform better in everything they do. I am an optimist and expect everyone around me to be. I expect my patients to come into the operating room with positive thinking. This allows me to perform better and I believe contributes to a successful outcome. Thinking positively decreases the release of our stress hormones that cause wear and tear on our bodies.

8. Decrease STRESS: As I stated above, I believe that stress does contribute to disease. When we are stressed, various chemicals in the body called hormones are released to help us deal and cope. These hormones, however, lower our bodies' defenses against infection, cancer and other diseases. There are many ways to deal with stress in our daily lives. I like to do yoga. Some people like to play golf. I also find that my exercise routine helps with my stress management. Some people like to meditate. I have even tried hypnosis and found it extremely relaxing. Whatever you like to do should be your time to relieve stress.

9. Spirituality: Whatever your beliefs may be, recent studies have shown that people who pray live longer. Maybe praying decreases stress and gives people a more positive attitude. One of the first studies on this subject was done in the 1980s by Randolph Byrd. He found that in a series

of hundreds of heart attack patients that those that prayed had significantly less complications.

A recent poll sponsored by the American Psychological Association revealed that 21% of Americans surveyed used "Praying/going to church/spiritual/meditation practices to cope with stress. This was second only to exercise (45%).

I believe that we are just beginning to understand these types of relationships in healing. A new approach that seems to be addressing some of these issues is called Integral Medicine. Integral Medicine looks beyond building from the best in standard health care, holistic and alternative approaches. Integral Medicine looks to examine health and healing as lifelong processes. Mind, body and spirit must interact in shaping our well-being.

10. Get regular check-ups: Certainly regular eye check-ups are vital for vision. Many eye problems that are treatable can be picked up by a routine exam. Like most problems, the earlier they are found, the more likely they will be treated successfully. Apply this to your general health as well.

Recent statistics have shown that about 64% of the Americans are overweight. That amounts to almost 130 million adults. The incidence of obesity has practically doubled since the 1960s. Obesity now rivals smoking as a major health risk. Although most of us are well aware of the health consequences obesity has on heart disease, high blood pressure, diabetes and cancer, recent research indicates that obesity puts people at risk for eye disease. It would appear that overweight individuals tend to consume less of the healthy types of foods. There have been studies to link poor nutrition to increased risk of macular degeneration. A higher incidence of cataract surgery has been found in patients with elevated blood pressure and cardiovascular (heart related) diseases. In addition, researchers have shown that an increase in body mass index strongly affects blood sugar levels, which is associated with an increased risk of cataract.

There has been a longstanding relationship between obesity and type 2 diabetes. Recent evidence has suggested that abdominal obesity may be a factor in retinopathy development. Remember that diabetic retinopathy can lead to blindness.

Also studies from Asia have found an association between elevated intraocular pressure, glaucoma and vascular disease. The authors conclude that obesity should be considered a risk factor for an increase in eye pressure. Interesting enough, there is evidence that patients who have glaucoma or are at risk of developing glaucoma can increase their intraocular pressure by 10% playing high resistance wind instruments (trumpet, oboe, French horn).

Vitamins and Eye Health

Not a day goes by in my practice that someone doesn't ask me about the role of vitamins and eye health. This is a very confusing topic because there is a lot of information available that is frequently not based on sound scientific data. My initial comment is that a sound diet should be the best and safest way to obtain an adequate supply of all requisite vitamins and minerals. That being said the following is a list of nutrients thought to be important for eye health and some potential sources. These are included under the category of **antioxidants**.

1. **Vitamin E: whole grain, nuts, vegetable oils (polyunsaturated) and olive oils (monounsaturated)**

2. **Vitamin C: citrus fruits, vegetables such as broccoli**

3. **Carotenoids (including luteins): fruits and dark leafy, yellow and green vegetables**

4. **Zinc: meat, poultry, fish and dairy products**

There is evidence from a large clinical trial called the Age Related Eye Disease Study (AREDS) that antioxidant supplements may benefit people with age related macular degeneration (AMD). Patients with intermediate or advanced stages of AMD had a lower rate of clinical progression that was clinically significant. The supplements used were vitamin E (400 IU), vitamin C (500 mg), beta-carotene (15mg), and zinc (80mg together with 2 mg of copper). Since these are higher doses than usually recommended, I always require my patients to fully discuss these supplements with their internists so as not to interfere with any other medications, including other vitamins.

Patients with a family history of AMD also frequently ask me whether taking the AREDS supplements makes sense. To date, there is no evidence to support beginning this therapy.

In these patients I just recommend a good daily multivitamin. There is no evidence, however, that the use of multivitamins slows the onset or progression of AMD. Since we are not absolutely sure, I don't believe it could hurt. There may be, however, a lower risk of cataract formation with multivitamin supplements. Recent studies have suggested that Vitamin C can help reduce the risk for certain forms of cataracts. The value of antioxidant supplements in preventing or slowing down diabetic retinopathy is unknown at this time. My best advice is that multivitamins should not be a replacement for a sound diet.

As of this writing, **lutein** has received much attention as a treatment for various eye disorders including AMD. Lutein is in the carotenoid family, like beta-carotene. Currently, the evidence is far from conclusive.

Herbal supplements have also been marketed extensively. **Bilberry** and **ginko biloba** are most talked about. Bilberry is promoted as improving night vision and ginko biloba supposedly increases blood flow (could be important in glaucoma management). To date, their effectiveness remains unsubstantiated in the scientific literature.

In closing, I would like to address one additional area that I feel is a major threat to our health, especially the eyes, the eyelids and the face. I am talking about the long-term effects of excessive sun exposure. I believe that there is enough evidence to suggest a contributory role of UV exposure in cataract and macular degeneration development. There is a definitive relationship between excessive sun exposure and skin cancer development. The sun plays a major role in aging the skin, causing photodamage (sunspots) and wrinkles. I recommend limiting sun exposure and always wearing sun block. This is easy to do and you will be surprised how much better your skin will age.

CHAPTER FOURTEEN

CONCLUSION

As I reflect back on my twenty years of practice, I consider it an honor and a privilege to have made a difference in so many people's lives. Whether it is restoring sight, removing a malignant tumor or cosmetically improving someone's appearance, being given this opportunity has more than fulfilled my life's goals.

In closing I would like to share with you a letter written by one of my patients, Diane W.

"January 1996, my husband died in my arms in our kitchen. In February I resumed my work as an X-Ray technician. While working the doctor's noticed I couldn't hear them well. That afternoon, they scheduled me for an MRI. Results came back as a benign brain tumor (acoustic neuroma). Surgery was performed in May leaving me with many residual conditions. Meningitis, a left upper lid gold implant, left facial paralysis, drooling, complete deafness of my left ear, severe imbalance causing constant nausea and short term memory loss. I THOUGHT MY LIFE WAS OVER….UNTIL in 1997 I met Dr. Kristan, Ophthalmic surgeon. Through numerous surgeries (Bleph's Nips and Tucks), this gifted man brought sunshine into my darkened life.

With his reconstructive surgery team, they have taken my miserable looking paralyzed face and turned it up and around to enjoy the warm sunshine again.

My heart wrenching tears and sobs have been exchanged for laughter and joy….For NOW I HAVE A LIFE ONCE MORE!!!

Due to my wonderful Dr. Kristan, my mentor (this man I consider Patron-Saint).

Again, thank you so much Dr. Kristan for your compassion, understanding, and Those God Gifted Perfect Surgical Hands. Where would I be today ----without you? "

God Blesses You through my Prayers
Diane W.

REFERENCE:

Seddon JM et al Progression of age-related macular degeneration: association with body mass index, waist circumference and waist-hip ratio Archives of Ophthalmology 2003; 121(6) pg 785

Lee JS et al Relationship between intraocular pressure and systemic health parameters in the Korean population Korean J Ophthalmology 2002; 16(1): pg 13

Van Leiden HA et al Blood pressure, lipids and obesity are associated with retinopathy: Diabetes Care 2002; 25(8) pg 1320

Mares JA et al Doctor, What Vitamins should I Take for My Eyes? Arch Ophthalmology 2004; Vol 122 Pg 628

Passo MS et al Exercise reduces intraocular pressure among subjects suspected of having glaucoma. Arch Ophthalmol 1991; 109 (8); 1096-1098

Aydin P et al Effect of wind instrument playing on intraocular pressure. J Glaucoma 2000:9:322-324

Appendix A
Pertinent Eyelid Anatomy

The eyelids and tissue around the eye constitute a very delicate and complex arrangement (Figure A). Beginning from the skin surface the layers of the eyelid from outside to inside are as follows.

The orbicularis muscle surrounds the eye in a circular fashion in both the upper and lower eyelids. The orbicularis muscle is responsible for closing the eye. The orbicularis muscle is therefore very important in the blink mechanism and closing the eye for protection.

In the upper lid is **the levator muscle.** The levator muscle begins deep behind the eye and fans out in the upper eyelid to eventually attach to the tarsal plate and skin. The levator muscle is primarily responsible for elevating the upper eyelid. As you can see two different muscles work to open and close the upper eyelid. Another muscle that has a small role in elevating the upper eyelid is **Muller's muscle.** This muscle becomes more important in patients with thyroid eyelid problems. In the lower eyelid, one finds the **capsulopalpebral fascia**, a retractor of the lower eyelid. This fascia is analogous to the levator muscle of the upper eyelid.

The tarsal plate is a cartilaginous structure that gives support to the upper and lower eyelids. It is only in a portion of the eyelid. Without the tarsus, the eyelid would be very floppy. Within the tarsal plate are many oil producing glands called **meibomian glands.** The meibomian glands serve a vital function in maintaining the proper moisture in the eye. A blockage in these glands to one of the most common eyelid infections called a chalazion. A chalazion is sometimes confused with a stye.

Attached to the tarsus is the **orbital septum.** The orbital septum is a fine membrane that inserts into the tarsus and the bony rim around the eye. This structure keeps the **orbital fat** from protruding and creating unsightly "bags". The orbital fat surrounds the eye and acts like a "shock absorber" to protect the eyeball in case of injury.

Lining the inside of the eyelid and in contact with the eyeball is the **conjunctiva.** The conjunctiva is called a mucous membrane because it provides lubricating functions for the eye and eyelid.

The two corners of the eyelid where the upper and lower eyelids meet are called the **canthi.** **The lateral canthus** is located at the outer corner and **the medial canthus** is located at the inner corner.

The eyelid margin is where the upper and lower eyelids "end". The eyelid margin goes from one canthus to the other and is located at the level of the eyelashes. The distance between the upper eyelid margin and the lower eyelid margin defines how "opened "the eye is. This is called **the palpebral fissure.**

The eyebrows have a number of muscles that work to depress and one basic elevator. **The corrugator and procerus muscles** primarily depress the brow. Simply speaking these muscles are located between the brows. The corrugator and procerus muscles are the main muscles treated with botox for glabellar frowns. The main elevator of the brow is **the frontal muscle.** Contraction of this muscle can cause excessive forehead lines and is frequently treated with botox.

Lacrimal System

The tear duct or lacrimal drainage system is composed of two small openings, one in the upper eyelid and one in the lower eyelid. These are located near the medial canthus and are called the **lacrimal punctum**. They are small openings in the lid and constitute the beginning of the drainage apparatus. From the puncta the tears enter a narrow tube called the **canaliculus**. The canaliculi from the upper lid and lower lid connect together and drain into a reservoir called the **lacrimal sac**. From the lacrimal sac, the tears drain down a bony canal (**nasolacrimal duct**) on the inside of the nose and eventually empty into the nose and are swallowed. All this happens without one being aware of the process.

Tears are produced by the lacrimal gland located under the upper eyelid in outer part above the lateral canthus. Tears therefore have to travel from the upper outer area of the eye to the inner or medial canthus in order to go down the drainage system. This is accomplished by the active contractions of the eyelid muscles with each blink. Thus the blink mechanism is very important to help distribute the tears.

Orbital Imaging
The orbit consists of the eyeball and the surrounding bone , the muscles and connective tissue around the eyeball, the nerves supplying the eye and face, and the blood vessels. Surrounding the orbit are the sinuses.

1. **Plain orbital x-rays:** this modality is infrequently used since the development of CT scanning

2. **CT scanning or computerized tomography:** this is probably the most commonly used x-ray and the most important advance in the evaluation and management of orbital disease. It is best for looking at the bony detail of the orbit. Its disadvantage is that CT scanning involves radiation. Contrast material is frequently given intravenously a complete study. CT is not the ideal test for soft tissue (muscles, nerves, fat and blood vessels) evaluation.

3. **Magnetic Resonance Imaging (MRI):** involves imaging using a magnetic field and not x-rays. MRI is usually a better test for soft tissue problems. The main limitation

to MRI is the fact the test requires one to lie on a narrow table in a confining tube. This is, however, improving with open units and units where you can stand now widely available.

Figure A

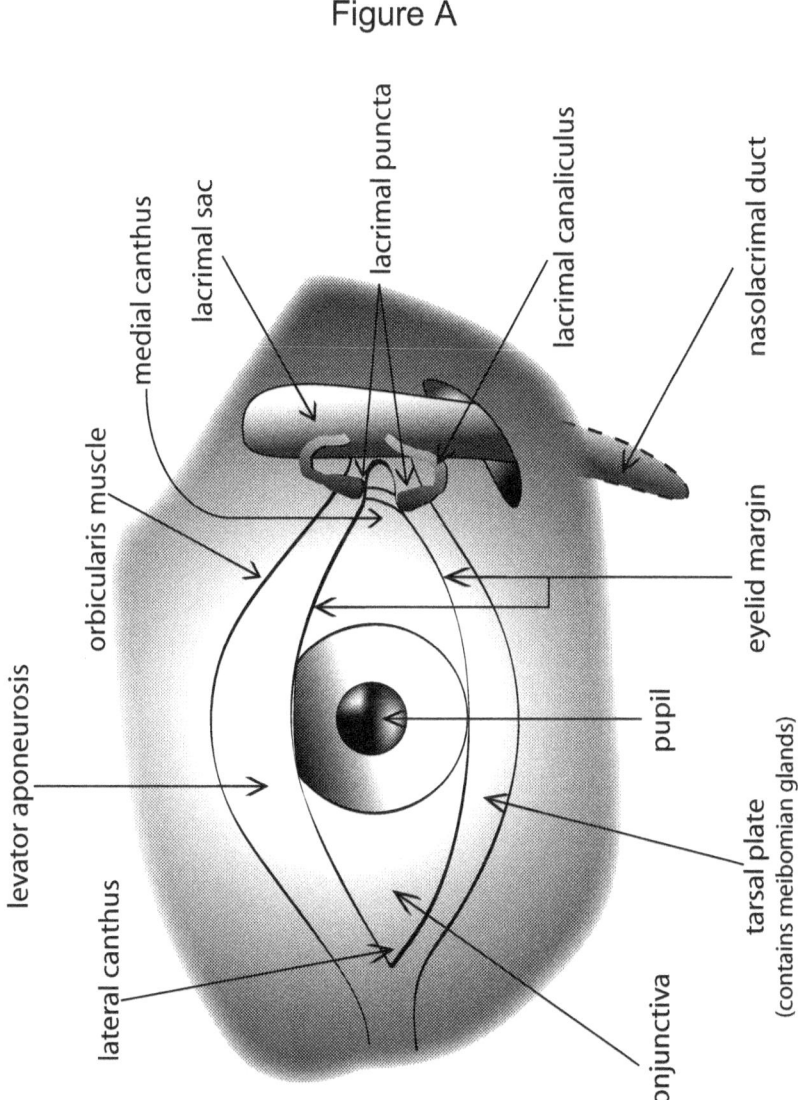

www.ingramcontent.com/pod-product-compliance
Lightning Source LLC
Chambersburg PA
CBHW022103170526
45157CB00004B/1462